HeartSmart
Nutrition

Shopping on the Run

Ramona Josephson RDN

Registered Dietitian and Nutritionist

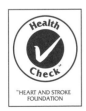

Health Check
HEART AND STROKE
FOUNDATION

Douglas & McIntyre
Vancouver/Toronto

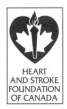

HEART
AND STROKE
FOUNDATION
OF CANADA

Douglas & McIntyre
2323 Quebec Street, Suite 201
Vancouver, British Columbia
V5T 4S7
www.douglas-mcintyre.com

National Library of Canada Cataloguing in Publication Data

Josephson, Ramona
    Heartsmart nutrition : shopping on the run / Ramona Josephson.
—Rev. ed.

    Includes index.
    Copublished by: Heart and Stroke Foundation of Canada.
    Previous eds. have title: The heartsmart shopper.
    ISBN 1-55054-983-9

    1. Nutrition. 2. Low-fat diet. 3. Grocery shopping. I. Heart and Stroke Foundation of Canada. II. Josephson, Ramona. Heartsmart shopper. III. Title.
TX356.J68 2003   613.2   C2003-910056-1

Editing by Elizabeth Wilson and Lucy Kenward
Copy-editing by Robin Van Heck
Cover and text design by DesignGeist
Illustrations by Hermani & Sorrentino Design
Printed and bound in Canada by Friesens
Printed on acid-free paper

The publisher gratefully acknowledges the financial support of the Canada Council for the Arts, the British Columbia Arts Council, and the Government of Canada through the Book Publishing Industry Development Program (BPIDP) for its publishing activities.

Contents

Foreword

For almost 50 years, unwavering public support has enabled the Heart and Stroke Foundation to continually invest and lead in the area of heart disease and stroke research and health promotion in Canada. The Foundation is constantly in search of programs and materials that can make a difference to people at risk, patients, their families and the general public. The Foundation develops these programs and materials to help empower you to make heart-healthy choices.

We know that small, everyday changes to your lifestyle can make a big difference to your overall health. Yet sometimes it seems so difficult to know where to start.

This third edition of *HeartSmart Nutrition: Shopping on the Run* offers very practical advice, including the latest information on nutrition labelling, as well as ideas on how to control your weight. Author and dietitian Ramona Josephson offers innovative ways to control your fat intake with the use of the old-fashioned teaspoon as a guide. This simple tip makes it easier than ever to choose healthy alternatives. Don't hesitate to use the book when you build your shopping list. Or better yet, take it with you to the grocery store.

Based on *Canada's Food Guide to Healthy Eating*, the book helps you use your shopping cart as a nutritional indicator in an unforgettable way. The book's illustrations and icons add to this by transforming nutrition principles into easily remembered bits of information.

HeartSmart Nutrition also provides you with information on the Foundation's flagship health promotion program, Health Check™. Health Check is an on-pack food information program that can help you make wise food choices at the grocery store. Health Check will help you interpret all of the nutrition information you now find on food packages. When you see the Health Check logo you know you are making a healthy choice.

The Heart and Stroke Foundation of Canada is committed to improving consumers' knowledge of nutrition and eating practices. *HeartSmart Nutrition: Shopping on the Run* and the Health Check Program are simple tools to help you make wise decisions about the foods you eat.

To your good health!

Carolyn Brooks

Carolyn Brooks
President
Heart and Stroke Foundation of Canada

Preface and Acknowledgments

Eating well does make a difference. I learned that firsthand as a teenager. My family has a strong history of heart disease, and we were devastated when my father was diagnosed with high blood cholesterol. At that time the role that diet might play in preventing this disease was just emerging. With typical determination my mother set out to change the family diet. Six months later my father's blood cholesterol was normal, we had all lost weight—and we felt great! I wanted to stand on the rooftops and tell the world: *If we can do it, you can too!* My parents have always remained my role models. They've led active lives, taken good care of their health and eaten the heart-healthy way. They planted the seed for my desire to "spread the word."

HeartSmart Nutrition was written with the love and support of my wonderful husband, Ken Karasick. My two kids, Jaclyn and Marc, are now at university and their interest in nutrition inspires me. My daughter and her roommate buy and prepare food the HeartSmart way. My son's friends discuss which is the healthiest bread. I realize that walking the talk *can* make a difference.

I would like to thank the following people who contributed their professional expertise, enthusiasm and creativity to the book. From the Heart and Stroke Foundation of Canada: Doug MacQuarrie, Director, Health Promotion; Carol Dombrow, Consultant Registered Dietitian; and the Health Promotion Initiative Review Committee and staff. From the Heart and Stroke Foundation of BC and Yukon: Richard Rees, former Executive Director and Fiona Ahrens, former Director, Marketing and Communications. My creative team included Angela Murrills, writing support; Michela Sorrentino, illustrations; Peter Cocking and Gabi Proctor, cover and text design; and Lucy Kenward and Elizabeth Wilson, editors. This book reflects the spirit and enthusiasm that went into it—fun, coordinated and user-friendly.

The hardest group to satisfy is one's peers and once again I put mine to the test, asking many of them to review all or part of the book. Thanks to my colleagues for your detailed analysis of the contents: Carol Dombrow, consultant to the Heart and Stroke Foundation of Canada; Garima Dwivedi, Nutrition Advisor, Office of Nutrition Policy and Promotion, Health Canada; Frances Johnson, Manager, Clinical Nutrition, St. Paul's Hospital, Vancouver; Susan Firus and Donna Forsyth, Dial-a-Dietitian of B.C.

And, of course, thanks again to Scott McIntyre of Douglas and McIntyre and his team of enthusiastic staff for acknowledging the value of HeartSmart nutrition by publishing this third edition!

INTRODUCTION

It's been five years since I wrote the first edition of this book. I've received hundreds of comments from people across Canada telling me how useful the book is in helping them make healthy choices daily. I had no idea it would become a Canadian bestseller. Doctors "prescribe" it. Colleagues recommend it to their patients in hospitals and clinics. People buy copies for their friends. It's a testament to the fact that Canadians are interested in what they eat, but find much of the information out there confusing. They want the facts in a way that is easy to digest.

Since the first edition much has happened. The good news is that Health Canada has come out with new food labelling laws that can help us make wise choices. At the same time, we have been deluged with so much *more* information. Sensationalized weight-loss diets, new and improved food products, cutting-edge research. These days there's even *more* to be confused about!

Discovering how to "read" these new labels is just part of what you'll find in this new edition. You'll also learn how to manage your weight without dieting. And how to use the information we are learning in current nutrition research. In short, you'll soon be in the express lane to healthy eating and weight control, the HeartSmart™ way.

Our journey begins in the supermarket with a simple concept called "shopping cart" shopping. In just three steps you'll learn the secret of a well-balanced diet. Guaranteed. You'll discover the simple "teaspoon solution" to fat budgeting that is key to managing calories. Visual icons lead you to HeartSmart ideas, Label Smarts and All Star Tips, answer frequently asked questions and offer Kidstuff and Penny Wise suggestions.

Making simple everyday heart-healthy choices can make a big difference to your health. In my nutrition coaching practice in Vancouver, I am constantly inspired by the vitality my clients experience as they achieve their personal nutrition goals. This book will show you that managing your weight and heart health is NOT about dieting and deprivation. And it's not an end in itself. It's a lifelong journey. One I hope you will enjoy.

Join me and the Heart and Stroke Foundation of Canada as you discover how to balance good nutrition with your hectic life, use your shopping cart as your nutrition barometer and enjoy all foods in balance!

Ramona Josephson

Ramona Josephson
RDN B.Sc. Hons. Dip. Ther. Diet
www.yournutritioncoach.com

DAILY B.R.E.A.D.

Too hard to remember heart health risk factors?
Not with this daily slice of B.R.E.A.D.

B **Blood Pressure and Blood Cholesterol** Do you know your numbers? High blood pressure and high blood cholesterol are risk factors for heart disease and stroke. They are silent conditions—but can be controlled by healthy living and/or by medication.

R **Relaxation** Have you stopped to smell the roses today? Let's face it, our harried lives leave much to be desired. It's not the stress that's the problem—today that's a given. It's how we deal with it that counts. Stress is a risk factor for heart disease, so take a few moments to breathe deeply and relax.

E **Eating Well** Do you? Obesity is a risk factor for heart disease. And most Canadians eat more fat and less fibre than is desirable. It's not for lack of choice. We're surrounded by choices—to buy, prepare and enjoy heart-healthy foods. It's about balance. The wise choice is yours for the taking.

A **Active Living** Are you moving? Activity is a prescription for an endless array of healthy outcomes. It decreases your risk for heart disease, reduces blood pressure and stress levels, helps you manage your weight, and makes you feel great. So remember, every day, to move a little, and then to move a little more.

D **Don't Smoke** A pack-a-day smoker has twice the risk for heart disease and stroke as a nonsmoker. And imagine this—each cigarette burns for 12 minutes, and during that time the smoker inhales for a mere 30 seconds. Meanwhile, chemicals are given off into the air and many are known causes of cancer. This is what nonsmokers breathe. So if you do, think D—Don't smoke! For all our sakes.

Make every day another healthy slice of life

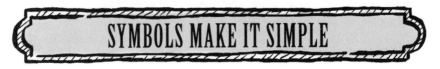
These simple symbols add up to a recipe for HeartSmart nutrition.

Reading a book on nutrition can be like eating a 12-course dinner without a break. You get indigestion! That's why I've broken the information down into bite-sized pieces and highlighted them with a system of icons—symbols— that help to make each point memorable and simple to use. All together, they add up to a recipe for HeartSmart™ nutrition.

Here's the central concept of this book; it's the express lane to sensible nutrition. Starting on page 5, you'll learn to separate your shopping cart into 1-2-3 parts and remember which food groups belong where. When you've got the idea you'll discover it's fun and easy. As the Health Check™ program grows (see page 140), food choices will become even easier—and you'll become a HeartSmart shopper for life.

Find out how to shop for vitamins, minerals, phyto-chemicals and antioxidants by choosing foods high in these nutrients.

At last! Canada has mandatory nutrition labelling. These tips will tell you how to use the information on labels to select a healthy diet.

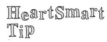

These are simple and heart-healthy ways to modify your daily diet to make it HeartSmart. The term "HeartSmart" incorporates the fat, fibre and sodium guidelines adopted by the Heart and Stroke Foundation that reflect Health Canada's Nutrition Recommendations and Canada's Food Guide to Healthy Eating. A HeartSmart idea always meets these standards, whether as a nutrition tip in this book or a recipe in the Foundation's highly acclaimed cookbooks (for a list, see page 150).

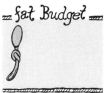

Using the teaspoon solution, you'll find out how to make smart fat-budgeting decisions for yourself and your family as you whiz through the supermarket. Just remember, 1 teaspoon of fat = approximately 5 grams. And some fats are better than others.

These are quick and easy tips to use on a daily basis to boost nutrition—and make *you* a star!

Discover interesting tidbits of information about the foods we eat, food trends and food history. Great to share with friends and family.

Confused about nutrition? I've tried to answer the most common questions. You can also check the Appendix or ask the Heart and Stroke Foundation.

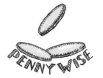

Here you'll find old-fashioned frugality. Find out how to get the most nutrition for your money by following these foolproof buying, storing and cooking tips.

Simple tips about nutritious foods that kids will love—and you'll feel good about giving them. Great ideas for grown-ups too.

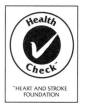

This growing not-for-profit food information program from the Heart and Stroke Foundation of Canada will make wise food choices even easier. A Health Check logo on the package tells you that the product has been reviewed by the Heart and Stroke Foundation and is part of healthy eating. See page 140 for details.

NUTRITION 1-2-3

Organize your shopping cart the way Canada's Food Guide to Healthy Eating organizes food groups for good nutrition.

Eating well can be easy—and here's the proof.

We are surrounded by choices. Some are HeartSmart™ whereas others are not. Knowing the difference is the key. In this little book, I cut through the confusion and give you the simple facts. You discover how to use tools not rules to achieve a healthy weight and to eat the HeartSmart way. And that means your way. We are all different in our likes and dislikes, and no one diet fits us all. Eating well is about variety, options and choice—your choice. I'll show you how.

Our journey begins in the supermarket.

In the next few pages, I'll show you how to shop nutritiously for the rest of your life. Honest!

One simple idea. Organize your shopping cart the same way that Canada's Food Guide to Healthy Eating organizes food groups for good nutrition. That's it! Sound too easy? Read on.

Nutrition 101 made super simple

The foods we eat contain over 50 different nutrients, each with a story to tell. It seems impossible to remember them all.

Canada's Food Guide to Healthy Eating cuts through the clutter. It's been designed by experts who've spent hours poring over technical literature to structure a diet that will help us stay healthy. The guide groups foods that contain similar, but not identical nutrients, and places them on the bands of the familiar rainbow to illustrate how much of each group we should choose.

According to Canada's Food Guide to Healthy Eating:

The key to good nutrition is to balance a variety of foods from each group and consume them in the appropriate quantities. How do we do that?

- Make more choices from the two outer bands of the rainbow: the grain products, and vegetables and fruit.
- Make fewer choices from the two inner bands of the rainbow: the milk products, and meat and alternatives.
- Be cautious about our choices from the foods not listed on the rainbow: the fats, oils and others. These also fit, but remember, it's all about balance.

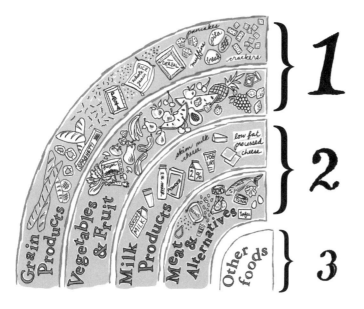

Introducing (tah-dah!)
The HeartSmart Shopping Cart

The rainbow is handy, but it's even simpler and more practical to use a universal food guide: the shopping cart. You see it every time you go to the store. I want you to see it now in a totally different way, so that by the end of this book your shopping cart will become the guide to your nutrition choices. It's that simple.

Easy as 1-2-3

Your shopping cart has three parts:

Let your cart be your guide

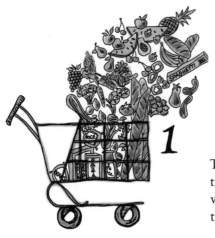

Think Big. Think the two outer bands of the rainbow. Pick whole-grain products, vegetables and fruit in abundance to fill the big part of your cart.

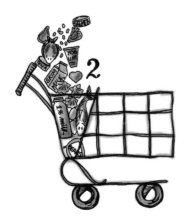

Think Smaller. Think the two inner bands of the rainbow. Use the #2 part to help you choose milk products, meat and alternatives more deliberately.

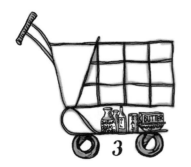

Think Lower. Select your fats, oils and others carefully and put them here.

Nutrition 201

Why to choose plant foods in abundance

- They're mostly made of complex carbohydrates and fibre our bodies need.
- Most contain so little fat that you can forget about it.
- They contain no dietary cholesterol.
- They're loaded with vitamins, minerals, antioxidants and phytochemicals (more about these later…).

So go ahead! Fill the big #1 part of your cart to your heart's content. Load it up with high-fibre cereals, breads, grains, veggies and fruit.

Plants are our main source of fibre, and experts recommend that we increase the amount of fibre that we eat. Fibre helps keep us regular, may help prevent bowel diseases and has been connected with the prevention of heart disease, diabetes and some cancers. For more information, see page 42.

Why to be deliberate with animal foods

The two inner bands of the rainbow contain mostly foods that come directly or indirectly from animals and seafood. Milk products, meat, poultry and fish belong here. These foods are clustered together because they all provide protein. Many are sources of iron—in a form more readily absorbed than from plant foods—and calcium, zinc and vitamin B12.

But they all contain dietary cholesterol and many contain fat—and often saturated fat—both of which we should try to reduce in our diets.

You'll learn how to make healthy lower-fat choices and to enjoy these foods in moderation. Be deliberate about how you fill the smaller #2 part of your cart, choosing lower-fat milk products, leaner meat, fish and legumes—an easy way to stay within your fat budget.

Meats contain *no* fibre. Fibre is found *only* in plant cells.

Plants contain *no* dietary cholesterol. Cholesterol is found *only* in animal cells.

Why are legumes in this part of the cart?
Canada's Food Guide to Healthy Eating places legumes—dried peas, beans and lentils—with meat and alternatives because they are high in protein. But they could be in the #1 part of the cart. Like other plants they are high in fibre, low in fat (except soybeans) and contain no cholesterol. No need to limit these!

Why to choose fats, oils and others...carefully

Fats and oils are an integral part of our diet, but most of us eat too much or have trouble making wise choices. Many of the foods they are added to are not on the rainbow because they don't offer enough nutritional value relative to their high fat content.

Keeping this "lower" group in balance can be our biggest challenge. You will find out how to separate the issues of quantity and quality of fats and oils, so that you can think carefully about what you add to the lower part of your cart. Aim to keep quantities small.

Psst...placing a shopping basket under your cart will prevent #3 items falling off, and remind you to "contain" what you're buying.

Moms and dads...is the #2 part of the cart where you place your child? Use a shopping basket in the #1 part for your #2 foods.

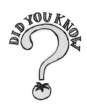

Here's how to read the rainbow with care.

Plant foods: the rainbow does not distinguish between high-fibre and low-fibre carbohydrates. Refined carbohydrates are stripped of many nutrients; they can cause spikes in blood sugar and lead to overindulging. Choose whole grains whenever possible.

Animal foods: the rainbow does not distinguish between lower- and higher-fat milk products or lean and fatty meats. Less fat is better.

Fats and oils: all fats are calorie-dense. Keep quantities small—and always remember, unsaturated fats are a healthier choice.

Top nutrition at top speed

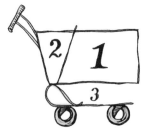

1. Feel free to fill the big #1 part of your cart, loading it up with grains, veggies and fruit.
2. Be deliberate about how you fill the smaller #2 part of your cart, choosing lower-fat milk products, leaner meat, fish and legumes.
3. Think carefully about everything you add to the #3 lower part of your cart.

THE HEARTSMART SHOPPING LIST

Write your shopping list the same way you fill the parts of your cart and you'll provide your family with variety and balance.

Grab a piece of paper and imagine it's divided into three unequal parts. Fold the page in half from top to bottom. Open it out and then fold the bottom half in to a third of its depth. Write #1, #2 and #3 on the three sections like this:

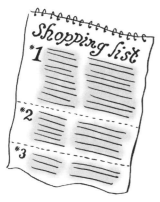

1 Big! Load up—with grains, vegetables and fruit.

2 Smaller! Be deliberate—choose lower-fat milk products, leaner meats, fish and legumes.

3 Lower! Think carefully—limit fats, oils and others.

As you write down what you plan to buy, you reinforce your nutrition savvy by allocating those foods to the #1, #2 and #3 parts of your list because the list reflects the way you fill your shopping cart.

After you've written your list, ask yourself, *Have I included enough whole grains, veggies and fruit? Did I choose lower-fat milk products, and are there enough of them? Did I select a range of lower-fat meats, fish and legumes?* Last of all ask yourself, *Did I think carefully about fats, oils and others— are there too many?* Maybe you'll need to revise your list.

With this list in your hand, you'll whiz through the aisles, secure in the knowledge that even on the run you're a HeartSmart™ shopper.

• Avoid going to the store when you're hungry. If you've got the growlies, it's all too easy to make impulsive choices.

• Leave your shopping list on the fridge. As you and your family add to it, you'll reinforce the importance of the food groups and how to establish healthy, balanced eating habits.

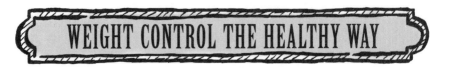
Managing your weight is making simple changes you can live with. You're already on your way.

Canadians spend millions of dollars every year on weight-loss diets and gimmicks, yet as a nation we are still gaining weight. There **is** a better way.

Managing your weight is not dieting or deprivation. It's making simple changes that you can live with. It's achieving your healthy weight with the very same foods that you'll continue to eat after you've lost that weight. The key is to pay more attention to what you choose, when you eat and how much. And to move a little more, a little more often.

You've read about top nutrition at top speed. You're ready to load up your HeartSmart™ shopping cart with foods that will give you the nutrients and energy you need to be healthy. Congratulations. You're now on your way to developing a weight management plan you can live with.

What's a healthy weight?

Don't even compare yourself with those computer-manipulated cover models! Great bodies come in all sizes and shapes. Weight control the healthy way means achieving your healthiest weight—and there's quite a range. Check the chart on page 145 to determine a healthy weight for your height. Being in the Health Risk Zone means you're at increased risk for heart disease, diabetes and stroke. Being underweight means an increased risk of osteoporosis.

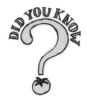

Are you an apple or a pear? "Apples" who carry weight around their waist are at greater risk of heart disease than "pears" who bear it around their hips. A waist measurement greater than 40 inches (102 cm) on a man and 35 inches (88 cm) on a woman may indicate higher health risks.

Your **best** weight loss strategy—**eat!**

Surprised? Read on.

Food is designed to give you energy and nourish your body. Fuel your tank the right way. Skipping meals or going for hours without food is like running on empty. Your body can stall too, just like a car. Keep it fuelled and it keeps on going. When you supply your body with energy throughout the day, your metabolic rate stays up, you feel more energetic and you're less inclined to dive for the fridge. That need for a quick fix is driven by the slump in your blood sugar. Why set up this situation? Instead, get in touch with your body's real needs and take control of your food choices.

Serving **size**—how **much** is enough?

People's energy needs vary widely. Usually, the larger your build and the more active you are, the more portions you can eat. Below, you will find a quick and easy guide. For health's sake, women should eat at least the minimum number of servings from all of the bands of the rainbow, men a little more.

Develop a feel for a serving size by visualizing the quantity of a typical food in each band of the rainbow. Here's an easy guide:

	Typical one-serving size	Number of servings in a day
Grains	1 slice of bread or 1/2 cup rice	5–12
Fruit	size of a tennis ball	5–10
Veggies	1/2 cup cooked or 1 cup raw	
Milk	1 cup	2 or more
Meat	size of a deck of cards	2–3
Fat	1 tsp oil	3–6 tsp

• Choose foods high in fibre such as whole grains, fruits, vegetables and legumes. They take longer to chew and fill you up more than refined foods.
• Choose leaner meats and lower-fat milk products. The less fat the better.

Meal Planning Made Easy

Plan meals to give you continuous energy, with the right balance of nutrients.

Ask yourself these three questions about what you're planning to put on your plate:

1. *Where is the protein?* Protein is essential as it provides several hours of satiety (it keeps you feeling full longer). Choose proteins that are low in saturated fats from the #2 part of your cart. Try lower-fat milk products, chicken or turkey breasts, fish, lean meat, legumes.

2. *What is the carbohydrate?* Go for the highest-fibre source for added satiety, as well as nutrients. You'll find carbohydrates in the #1 part of your cart. Avoid refined carbohydrates, which are a quick fix and do not sustain you.

3. *How much is fat?* Use small amounts of unsaturated fats; limit your saturated fats. Fats make you feel full for longer—but they have the most calories. Some fat is a good idea, but less is still better. Find out how to make the best choices as you load up the #3 part of your cart.

The Power of the Plate

Divide your plate in half. Fill one half with veggies or salads. Divide the other half in two—one quarter for the protein, the other for the grain or starchy vegetable.

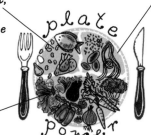

• Choose leaner meat, poultry or fish that's roughly the size of the palm of your hand.

• Add a higher-fibre grain that's about the size of your fist.

• Load up with veggies. Super-size them.

• Sprinkle or cook your food with a small amount of unsaturated fat, such as nuts, olive oil, canola oil. See Mighty Meals, page 125.

A healthy rate of weight loss is 1 to 2 pounds per week.

Snacking is a must

If meals are more than 4–5 hours apart, snacking is a must—even if you're not hungry. Many people feel the subtle signs of low blood sugar—dull headaches, tiredness—but put them down to it being just "that time of day." In fact your body is telling you that your blood sugar is dropping. Other people don't feel the low, but find themselves eating too much, too fast by the next meal time. A small low-calorie snack such as a fruit, low-fat yogurt or low-fat latte is all it takes to keep your energy level—and to keep you in control of your choices.

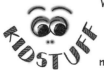 When the kids roar in from school, they're usually famished. They'll eat whatever is around. What better time to teach them good nutrition habits by eating your healthy mid-afternoon snack with them. Be a role model. Actions speak louder than words.

Here are some tips:

- Set out freshly cut fruit. You'll be surprised how much fruit gets consumed when it's out in the open.
- Put out low-fat, whole-grain crackers and peanut butter, rice cakes or low-fat yogurts. These snacks are good for the kids—and for you.
- Pack your fridge with cut-up veggies and lower-fat dips; buy them ready-made if time is short.
- Let kids buzz their own fruit smoothies.
- Limit temptation. Keep cookies in a high cupboard or don't buy them. Out of sight, out of mind.
- For more ideas, see Simple Snacks, page 130.

Make a meal that keeps on going

Yes, life is increasingly hectic. But set aside at least 15 minutes to enjoy your meal. That's how long it takes for your brain to register that you have eaten. Eat too fast and your brain does not "know" that you are full so you start to look for more to eat—usually that high-fat chocolate chip cookie.

Try this instead. Eating a sandwich for lunch? Make it big with lettuce, cucumber and tomato, so it takes longer to chew. Add veggie sticks on the side—celery, peppers, carrots. It will now take even longer to eat. You add very few extra calories, yet you walk away from the meal feeling more satisfied. Your body will thank you too—you've just fuelled it with phyto-chemicals and antioxidants.

I want to see results quickly. What is the best way?
If you just want to drop weight fast, any diet will work. But... slow down! Almost any diet will make you lose weight because you're consuming fewer calories overall. Conventional diets are like a light switch. You're either "on" them or "off" them. However, a diet designed only to achieve weight loss without thinking about health or sustainability is not a healthy diet. And it invariably leads to weight gain when you go off it.

Managing your weight sensibly means using the very same foods that you'll continue to eat after you've lost the weight.

Drop 90 pounds overnight... guaranteed!!!!!! Is it possible?
Gotcha. When you want to lose weight, you're ready to believe anything. Should you go high fat, low carbohydrate, high carbohydrate, low fat, high protein, low protein? No wonder so many of us are confused.

About carbs—the highs and lows

The low-carbohydrate diet, also known as "the high-protein, high-fat diet," is the latest craze. It lets you eat as much protein and fat as you like, as long as you limit carbohydrates. If that doesn't sound healthy, that's because it's not.

It is low in plant foods, all those foods in the #1 part of your cart. By all means cut down on refined carbohydrates, such as white breads and bagels and refined pastas, which are stripped of so many nutrients. But don't cut down on plant foods and whole grains.

Eating carbohydrates the HeartSmart way means you can lose weight AND enjoy the health benefits. Nutrients in high-fibre grains and plants offer protection against heart disease, diabetes, cancer and constipation. Plant foods add a gorgeous array of textures, colours, shapes and flavours to your diet. And including foods lower on the food chain is environmentally friendly.

Q&A *Why is it so often said that a "high-carbohydrate, low-fat diet" does not lead to weight loss?*

Because it has been taken too literally! The mantra: "Eat a diet high in carbohydrates and low in fat" has been interpreted to mean eat as much as you like as long as it is fat-free. And Canadians did. But sadly, calories do not magically disappear in the absence of fat. Eating too much of anything leads to weight gain. Recommended daily servings (see page 11) can add up quickly. One large bagel can equal three to four servings of grains. A plate (2 cups) of pasta is four servings! A high-carbohydrate diet is not an invitation to indulge. Carbohydrates count: eat whole grains—to give your body the health benefits that they provide.

About fat—the basics

We all need some fat in our diet. It's eating too much of it that's the problem. You may be consuming a lot more fat than you realize. Choosing lower-fat options reduces your calorie intake without compromising your health.

Why budget fat? Because fat is our most "fattening" nutrient! It provides more than twice the energy or calories of carbohydrates and protein. Some fat is OK. It's too much that's the problem.

1 gram carbohydrate	=	4 calories
1 gram protein	=	4 calories
1 gram fat	=	9 calories

The fat we eat may already be a natural part of a food, such as cheese. Fat may also be blended into food during its preparation—muffins are one example. It may be added to our food too, as in salad dressings. In fact each of the four food groups includes foods that may contain fat. Being aware of where fat shows up in your food will help you decide how to spend your fat budget.

Budgeting your fat is so important in managing weight and maintaining good health that I'll show you how to do it, step by step, in the next chapter.

Less is not better!

It sounds logical. If more calories = more weight gain, fewer calories = more weight loss. Right? Only up to a point.

Even when you are asleep, your body is busy. Your heart continues to beat, your lungs expand and contract, your cells manufacture essential chemicals, and so forth. The rate at which your body burns energy to maintain these functions is called your *basal metabolic rate,* or BMR.

If you eat fewer calories than you need to maintain your BMR, your body functions more slowly to use up less energy. It's a survival technique. With a low-calorie diet, you might lose weight quickly initially but, with your BMR slowed down, it's easy to gain it back—and more—when you go back to your old eating habits. Even worse, you gain back fat tissue rather than muscle. This makes it harder to lose weight again, because fat tissue burns energy more slowly. The result? You end up fighting your body instead of nurturing it.

Your best weight loss strategy—eat the healthy way

Eat regularly and eat before you get really hungry! Eat a healthy snack between meals to maintain your blood sugar level. You don't need to spend hours preparing a meal: you'll find simple recipes for One-minute Breakfasts, Power Lunch bags and Dinners in a Dash in the Mighty Meals chapter on page 125.

Don't try to change your eating habits all at once. Take one step at a time. Practise. Soon this new way of eating will become so natural that you won't even notice the change. Again and again my clients tell me "I don't even feel like I'm on a diet yet the kilos keep coming off. And I feel great!" This is a real lifestyle change you can live with.

Drink lots of fluid—at least eight glasses a day. Beverages containing caffeine don't count. Coffee, black tea, colas and alcohol all cause the body to lose fluid.

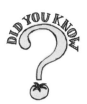

Alcohol does not appear on the rainbow, but it does count!
- A glass of red wine a day may be a recommendation for heart health, but remember—alcohol has calories, it encourages fat storage and it might increase your appetite.
- Choosing a mixed drink? Avoid the extra calories in the added tonic or cola. Try it with ice water or soda water instead.
- Enjoy white wine? Add soda and a wedge of lime to reduce the calories.

Move a little, Move a little more often

You can increase your basal metabolic rate by moving more. Activity shifts your body composition to more lean tissue and less fat tissue. Lean tissue burns more calories, whether you're walking, cleaning the house or even sleeping. Smart.

Moving your body means active living as well as planned exercise. Use the stairs instead of the elevator, park the car at the far end of the parking lot, meet your friends for a "walk break" rather than a coffee break. Small steps add up!

People who are overweight tend to be much less active than people who aren't.

As you increase muscle tone, you will look trimmer than your weight on the scale may indicate.

Weight loss at a glance

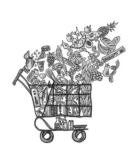

1. Eat! Enjoy the wonderful array of choices across the rainbow.
2. Plan healthy meals and snacks.
3. Watch your portion sizes.
4. Budget your fat intake.
5. Increase your activity.

Snapshot of a healthy day

Enjoy the wonderful array of choices across the rainbow, and watch your portion sizes.

Breakfast WHOLE-GRAIN CEREAL OR OAT BRAN WITH LOW-FAT MILK AND FRUIT

CEREAL: Start your day with a high-fibre cereal to keep hunger at bay throughout the morning. Oat bran is high in soluble fibre, the type that helps lower blood cholesterol. Sprinkle with flaxseeds.

SKIM MILK: Choose milk with the lowest amount of fat possible. Enjoy skim milk with cereal and try 1% in your coffee or tea. Low-fat soymilk is a healthy alternative.

BANANA OR ORANGE: Add fruit to increase the fibre and antioxidants in your diet. A citrus fruit adds vitamin C, which boosts iron absorption.

Lunch TURKEY OR CHICKEN BREAST SANDWICH WITH A SIDE OF VEGETABLES

BREAD: Choose whole-grain breads, buns and bagels but watch the size.

SPREAD: Spread it thin. "White" spreads such as butter, margarine and mayonnaise are the highest-fat selections. Use lower-fat margarine or lower-fat/fat-free mayonnaise on one side only and add mustard, relish or cranberry sauce to spruce up the taste.

TURKEY OR CHICKEN: Opt for skinless turkey or chicken breast. Tuna and salmon, and veggie "ham" or "turkey" slices are good bets. Lean roast beef and ham are OK, too. Go very easy on processed meats such as sausages and corned beef, and high-fat cheeses. Avoid pre-packaged, fat-loaded tuna, egg and chicken salad sandwiches.

VEGETABLES: Load up your sandwich with lettuce, tomatoes, onions, cucumber, green peppers.

SIDE OF VEGETABLES: Enjoy raw vegetables such as carrots, peppers, broccoli, cauliflower, celery.

Snack　　　LOW-FAT LATTE OR YOGURT WITH A FRUIT

Have a mid-afternoon snack, even if you don't feel hungry. It'll help curb your appetite so that you're not famished by dinnertime.

Dinner　　　SESAME-GINGER SALMON WITH BROWN RICE, STEAMED VEGGIES AND A LARGE SALAD

SALMON: Vary your proteins. Choose skinless chicken or turkey breast, fish, lean meat, tofu or legumes. Make dinners in a dash, low in fat and high in flavour.

BROWN RICE: Choose brown over white for fibre, or tuck into a medley of root vegetables such as yams, sweet potatoes and potatoes.

VEGETABLES: Enjoy them steamed, stir-fried or microwaved. Use oil sprays for stir-fries. Roast with a little olive oil, garlic and herbs. Going for seconds? Choose more veggies.

SALAD: A great filler. Use low-fat salad dressing or a seasoned vinegar.

STILL HUNGRY? Have more veggies or salads; they're loaded with nutrition and low in calories.

Snack　　　A FRUIT OR A GLASS OF LOW-FAT MILK

Fruit is always a great choice. Or choose a low-fat yogurt with puréed fruit sauce or a glass of warmed low-fat milk.

FAT BUDGETING MADE EASY

Here's a simple technique to budget your fat intake— the teaspoon solution.

It's no secret—we're eating too much fat. Fats are a concentrated source of energy. Too much fat = increased risk of obesity, heart disease and diabetes. Most experts consider that the fat in our daily diet should equal no more than 30% of our total daily calories.

Fat 101—Quantity

A little fat is OK. In fact it's not just OK, it's necessary. The problem is, most of us eat too much. After 1919 our daily intake shot up from 27% to 40% of our daily calories. Wow! It's fortunately on the downturn now but we need to be vigilant. New guidelines are being proposed, but for heart health the food we eat should provide us with no more than 30% calories from fat. So what does this mean in everyday terms, and how much fat should you budget in a day?

The daily fat intake recommended for the average man and woman is represented in the following chart. (Refer to My Four Steps to Estimating Your Personal Fat Budget on page 145.)

	Calories/day	Grams of fat
Women, 19 to 74	1800–2000	65 or less
Men, 19 to 74	2300–3000	90 or less

This chart shows you how many grams of fat you should consume in a day. It's a useful guide if you're in the habit of reading labels or food composition books. But not all foods are labelled, and who has the time to read lists and charts?

So, how do you calculate your fat intake? It's as easy as the Teaspoon Solution: a visual way to budget your fat intake for the day.

Fat budget for a day
—the good old teaspoon

Here's a way to keep fat budgeting really simple. Visualize a teaspoon of fat. That teaspoon equals approximately 5 grams of fat.

1 tsp fat = approximately 5 grams of fat

Each time you sit down to eat a meal or snack, visualize the teaspoons of fat contained in what you are about to eat. Throughout this book, I have listed approximately how many teaspoons of fat are in many of the foods we eat. These are average amounts and are a useful guide to making HeartSmart decisions. Now, use the handy chart that follows to determine how many of those teaspoons you should budget in a day.

	Calories/day	Grams of fat	Teaspoons of Fat
Women, 19 to 74	1800–2000	65 or less	13 or less
Men, 19 to 74	2300–3000	90 or less	18 or less

If your personal goal is to lose weight you may find that targeting a daily diet with 20% to 25% total calories from fat is more desirable. Don't go lower—you need some fats for health.

Throughout the book I will show you how to budget your fat wisely, choosing healthier fats more often. As you use up your fat budget throughout the day, visualize how many teaspoons remain. When you shop, use the fat budget lists at the beginning of each chapter and make a mental note of the teaspoons of fat in your favourite food choices. You may be surprised to find many lower-fat options to enjoy.

Fat Budget

Change from this	to this	and save!
grain products (#1 part of the cart)		
1 medium muffin	1 multi-grain bagel	2 tsp fat
1 croissant	1 whole-grain bun	2 tsp fat
1 cup instant ramen noodles	1 cup wild rice	3 tsp fat
vegetables and fruit (#1 part of the cart)		
20 french fries	1 baked potato	4 tsp fat
1 slice apple pie	1 apple	3 tsp fat
milk and milk products (#2 part of the cart)		
1 cup (250 mL) homo milk	1 cup skim milk	2 tsp fat
1"x1"x3" (50 g) cheese	1 cup 2% cottage cheese	3 tsp fat
1/2 cup plain ice cream	1 cup no-fat yogurt	2 tsp fat
meat and alternatives (#2 part of the cart)		
3 1/2 oz (100 g) ribs	3 1/2 oz sirloin or flank steak	3 tsp fat
3 1/2 oz regular ground beef	3 1/2 oz extra lean ground beef	2 tsp fat
3 1/2 oz skinless white chicken	3 1/2 oz dark chicken with skin	2 1/2 tsp fat
fats, oils and others (#3 part of the cart)		
30 potato chips	3 cups air-popped popcorn	4 tsp fat
1 small chocolate bar	1 fruit	3 tsp fat
1 tbsp mayonnaise	1 tbsp fat-free mayonnaise	2 tsp fat
2 tsp margarine	2 tsp low-fat margarine	1 tsp fat

Decide for yourself how to spend your teaspoons of fat. Enjoy your favourite high-fat foods without guilt by planning ahead and including them as an occasional treat. Remember, all foods can fit into a healthy eating plan.

If I move more can I eat more? How much more?
Your fat budget and calorie requirements are dependent on your level of physical activity. Refer to My Four Steps to Estimating Your Personal Fat Budget on page 145.

I love the taste of fat. Will I ever stop craving it?

Yes, you CAN lose your craving for things you think you can't live without. Your body will adapt. Have you already changed from homo to a lower-fat milk? Remember how different it tasted in the beginning? Yet now you're probably used to it. Be consistent about the changes you make—once your body gets used to them, it will crave these healthier foods.

• Foods you buy are labelled with the fat represented in grams. Remember: 5 grams of fat = approximately 1 teaspoon fat. Divide the grams by 5 and you can see, as a general guideline, where a food fits into your fat-budgeting chart.

• Look for the Health Check™ logo on a growing number of food packages. Products that carry the Health Check logo are wise choices based on Canada's Food Guide to Healthy Eating.

Although fat budget goals don't apply to children who are still growing, children often need the calories of higher-fat foods to help them develop. Fat should be reduced gradually so that by the time they end puberty their fat intake is that of an adult. In the meantime, let them learn by example—yours—how to enjoy lower-fat foods.

Although you should try to consume no more than 30% of your calories from fat, you don't need to relate the 30% value to every individual food to see if it fits (see page 147). The 30% figure applies to your overall diet—what you eat daily or even weekly. Using the fat budget system you can balance lower-fat foods with higher-fat foods to meet your goal. A HeartSmart diet doesn't mean cutting fat out. It just means cutting down—and choosing foods carefully.

Fat budgeting at a glance

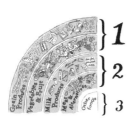

}**1**
}**2**
}**3**

Canada's Food Guide to Healthy Eating divides food into bands of a rainbow to highlight groups of foods abundant in similar nutrients. However some foods have too much fat relative to their nutritional content. Use the fat budget chart at the beginning of each "shopping cart" chapter to decide how to spend your fat budget to suit your needs.

Screech! Put the brakes on! Fat can be saturated, monounsaturated, polyun-saturated, hydrogenated or a trans fatty acid. What do they mean?? And how can a HeartSmart™ shopper make sense of them on the run? Read on…

Fat 201–Quality

Fat 101 was all about the quantity of fat. All fats have the same caloric value, but when it comes to heart health, not all fats are created equal. Different fats affect your body in different ways. Limit foods that contain saturated fat or hydrogenated fat.

Saturated fat AND hydrogenated fat are the ones to reduce

These fats raise blood cholesterol, so you should eat less of them. Saturated fat is found naturally in many foods, but it is also manufactured when unsaturated fat is processed. This is called hydrogenation, a process used to change liquid oils into a spreadable or solid form.

DID YOU KNOW

Saturated, monounsaturated and polyunsaturated fats (see Appendix, page 146, for definitions) appear in different combinations in different foods. So for instance, when we say that foods from animal sources contain saturated fats, it's not actually the whole story. In fact, they contain mostly saturated fatty acids.

Here's where you'll most often find saturated fat

- In the #2 part of your cart: whole-milk products and some meat products are high in saturated fats. This is why you need to budget fat wisely here.
- In the #3 part of your cart: the tropical vegetable oils are high in saturated fat. Watch out for palm, palm kernel and coconut oil on the labels of processed food. The less you choose the better.

Here's where you'll most often find hydrogenated fat

- In the #1 part of your cart: many baked goods use hydrogenated fat.
- In the #3 part of your cart: many products contain fats that are processed to harden them. Look out for the words "hydrogenated" or "partially hydrogenated" in the ingredient list and choose food with these ingredients less often.

When a fat is hydrogenated, the process creates saturated fat as well as trans fatty acids. Both fats raise blood cholesterol. Check the Nutrition Facts table and look for the product with the least of these fats.

- If it's a solid block (butter, lard, shortening or stick margarine) it's either saturated or hydrogenated.

- If it's liquid at room temperature (oil) it's unsaturated. Liquid is better.

Unsaturated fats are the ones to choose

There are two types of unsaturated fats:

Monounsaturated fats
These appear to have a beneficial effect on cholesterol, especially when eaten in place of saturated fat; they lower LDL (the "bad" cholesterol) without lowering HDL (the "good" cholesterol).

Polyunsaturated fats
There are two important types: omega-6 and omega-3. Omega-3 fats may be especially protective against heart disease.

Here's where you'll most often find unsaturated fat

- In the #1 part of your cart: surprise. Most plant foods are low in fat—the exceptions are avocados and olives, which are high in monounsaturated fat.
- In the #2 part of your cart: omega-3 fatty acids are found in fatty fish such as salmon, mackerel, herring and sardines.
- In the #3 part of your cart: most nuts and oils are high in unsaturated fats. Olive and canola oils contain monounsaturated fat. Omega-3 fats are found in ground flaxseed, flaxseed oil, soybean oil, canola oil and walnuts.

Fat choices at a glance

1. It's not only the quantity of fat that matters, it's the quality.
2. Cut down on saturated, hydrogenated and trans fats.
3. Choose monounsaturated and omega-3 fats more often.

SUPERMARKET SAVVY

Every choice you make, every old habit you break, can make a big difference to your family's health in the long run.

The grocery store doors slide apart and suddenly you're in a world of amazing foodstuffs and alluring choices. New products, exotic fruits and vegetables, different cuts of meat, poultry, fish and shellfish that you may never have seen before, herbs and seasonings from the world's four corners. Enticing signage and labels that shout *Buy Me!* All the opportunities you could imagine to make fabulous meals—and to tempt you away from HeartSmart™ nutrition. So where do you begin? How do you stay nutrition smart...on the run?

Filling a HeartSmart shopping cart can start with a research trip. Once you've read through this book, investing a single half-hour can pay lifelong dividends in terms of good nutrition.

I know, I know—it isn't the most exciting invitation you've ever had. But taking a new look at nutrition means looking at your supermarket in a different light.

There are over 25,000 items to choose from in large supermarkets. Each time you walk into one you have hundreds of decisions to make. And yet the average shopper usually takes just seconds to decide what to buy. Doing a little research during a quiet time at your usual store can help you shop just as quickly, but far more wisely.

Go through this book at home. I've tried to keep it simple because I want you to remember a few simple facts. Then put theory into practice at your supermarket. The first time, don't buy a single thing! Just go from aisle to aisle, look at your family's favourites and recall what you've read. After just this one research trip to the supermarket, you'll be amazed at how fast you can select wisely, and be nutrition and money wise!

Run each item through your nutrition scanner

Does it fit with what you're trying to achieve? Will it help you keep to your fat budget? Compared with similar products on the shelf, how does it stack up? Has it got more fibre? A healthier fat? Does it have more fat and salt than other nutrients? Soon you'll be answering these questions automatically as you make the best choices and tick off the items on your shopping list.

Every time you buy your groceries, you're investing in your family's long-term health. This is serious stuff. Every choice you make, every old habit you break can make a big difference to their health and yours in the long run.

Going eyeball to eyeball with the products on the shelf

Items that are displayed from the waist to eye level and above sell more. In fact, this is the most desirable space on the supermarket shelves. When you look below you will often find bargains and better deals. Adult cereals (such as the high-fibre ones) are placed on the top shelves. Kids' cereals—and other junior favourites such as cookies and fruit snacks—are often placed at your kids' eye level. Basic cereals that may have been on the market for years are often on the bottom shelf.

Why items are where they are

To entice you to buy! Standing in the checkout line is a bore. After you've read about the latest Elvis sighting, there's not much else to do...except shop. No wonder supermarkets stock this area with magazines, candies, batteries and other small impulse items.

Usually, the outer ring of the supermarket is where you'll find perishable foods: baked goods, fruits and vegetables, meats and the milk products. Staples, such as milk and eggs, are often right at the back of the store so that even if you're only popping in for some basics you'll find yourself walking by shelves of tempting items. Be careful!

Cross-merchandising means displaying two products together that go together. Salsa and taco chips. Fresh fish and tartar sauce. Lettuces and gourmet salad dressings. Pasta and pasta sauce. Convenient? Yes. But do a mental check as to how they fit into your HeartSmart shopping cart.

New products are often displayed at the end of the aisle because this is where you slow down to turn the corner.

And what can entice you more than the fragrance of the bakery or the smell of free samples?

TAKE A LOOK AT LABELS

Food package labels can be a wealth of information if you know what to look for.

Reduced in calories! Cholesterol free! No added sugar! Reading labels is the ultimate in window shopping. Labels are designed to attract our attention, but they can help you compare products and select foods for healthy eating. And now reading labels has become easier.

Ever turned over a package of crackers or cookies to find out what you were eating—and couldn't find any nutrition information? That will soon be a thing of the past! Health Canada has worked with consumer groups, provincial and territorial governments, voluntary health organizations, health professionals associations, literacy groups and the food industry to develop a new system for nutrition labelling. It is based on sound science and reflects consumers' best interests.

Consistent and easier to find, the new labels are a huge bonus for Canadian shoppers. They can help you make informed choices that help meet your healthy eating goals. They also encourage industry to produce food products consistent with these goals—it's a win-win situation. Look for the Label Smarts icon and tips throughout the book to find out how food labels can help you make healthy and informed choices. For reliable updated information, log on to Health Canada's nutrition labelling Web site at www.healthcanada.ca/nutritionlabelling.

 No one food is a panacea for good health, but some choices are better than others. Compare food labels to ensure you're making the best choices as you load up your shopping cart.

 The following foods will *not* carry Nutrition Facts tables:
- foods served or sold in restaurants, cafeterias and take-outs
- fresh fruit and vegetables
- raw single-ingredient meat and poultry (except when ground) and raw single-ingredient fish and seafood
- foods packaged at the store at the time of sale, for example, deli meats and cheeses
- food prepared and processed at a store and sold on-site, for example, bakery items, cooked meats
- products with extremely small amounts of all 13 core nutrients, such as coffee beans, tea leaves, spices, seasonings and food colourings

What's on the label? What does it mean and how do I use it?

1. The facts

These are found in the Nutrition Facts table and the ingredient list on the side or the back of the package. You'll find them on almost all pre-packaged products. They tell you the number of calories and the quantity of 13 core nutrients, and the list of ingredients in the product.

2. The nutrition claims

These are found on the front of the package. They may include claims that highlight a specific nutrient in the product or that reinforce the health benefits of the food. Advertised as part of a lifestyle to reduce the risk of developing a chronic disease such as heart disease or cancer, they are used at the discretion of the manufacturer but must follow regulated guidelines.

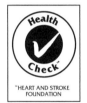

This symbol guides you to healthy choices. Look for it to make shopping even easier. Check out the details at: www.healthcheck.org.

Here are the Facts

1. The Nutrition Facts table

The Nutrition Facts table contains information on calories and 13 core nutrients. Its design is consistent (the same nutrients are listed in the same order) and user-friendly. Now it's easy to find, read and compare the nutrient content of similar foods. Once you are familiar with the Nutrition Facts table, you'll soon become a label expert.

Three reasons to use Nutrition Facts:

- to assess the calorie content of foods
- to compare similar or different types of foods
- to select foods that are high or low in specific nutrients

Serving Size

Under the Nutrition Facts heading, you'll find the description of a typical serving size. It's not a recommended serving! Compare the serving size to the amount of the food you usually eat at a sitting. If you consume more or less of the product, remember to adjust the nutrition facts accordingly.

Calories

The actual number of calories per serving from fat, carbohydrate and protein let you measure how much energy you'll get from that food. Everyone's caloric needs are unique; they vary by gender, age, body size and activity level. Remember: don't just look at the fat content of a food. It only reveals part of the picture.

Percentage of Daily Value

Health Canada identifies 13 core nutrients. The percentage of daily value lets you judge if there is a lot or little of the nutrient in a food serving. Values for calories and fat are based on a 2,000-calories-a-day diet and may differ depending on your individual energy needs.

It is optional to list the daily value for cholesterol because it is only of concern to those at risk for heart disease and diabetes.

There are no daily values for protein because most people get enough from a well-balanced diet, or for sugar because there is no acceptable targeted recommendation.

Carbohydrate

Also a source of energy, carbohydrates provide 4 calories per gram. Some carbohydrate foods are a source of dietary fibre. These are the ones to choose more often.

Fibre

There are two types of dietary fibre: soluble and insoluble. Although the label does not differentiate between the two, both are important. Soluble fibre helps to reduce blood cholesterol levels. Insoluble fibre plays a significant role in controlling and preventing bowel problems (see page 42). Most people need to consume more of both.

Protein

As a source of energy, protein provides 4 calories per gram. Protein forms the basis of all body tissues. Our muscles, organs, enzymes, antibodies and some hormones are made of protein.

Nutrition Facts
Per 1 cup (264g)

Amount	% Daily Value
Calories 260	
Fat 13g	**20%**
Saturated Fat 3g + Trans Fat 2g	**25%**
Cholesterol 30mg	
Sodium 660mg	**28%**
Carbohydrate 31g	**10%**
Fibre 0g	**0%**
Sugars 5g	
Protein 5g	
Vitamin A 4% • Vitamin C 2%	
Calcium 15% • Iron 4%	

Fat

A source of energy, fat provides the body with 9 calories per gram. Fat is an important part of your diet (see page 115), but most people eat too much. The Nutrition Facts table lists three numbers for fat: total fat, saturated fat and trans fat. These last two are the ones you want to choose less of. They are listed together because they have similar negative effects on your heart's health.

Saturated fats are found naturally in fats that are solid at room temperature, such as high-fat meat, milk products and tropical oils (see page 146).

Trans fats are created when vegetable oils are converted from liquid state to solid state (see page 146), a process called hydrogenation.

Cholesterol

Dietary cholesterol is found in all foods of animal origin. Eating more cholesterol may raise blood cholesterol levels, but eating more fat, especially saturated fat and trans fatty acids, is the main cause of high blood cholesterol.

Sodium

Sodium helps regulate water balance and blood pressure. In some people, sodium can elevate blood pressure. Check the labels on processed foods, which often contain more sodium than you realize. Sodium listed on the ingredient list has many names (see page 149).

Vitamins and minerals

Vitamins A and C, and the minerals calcium and iron are listed because of their potential health benefits.

VITAMIN A: for vision, to help form and maintain healthy skin, teeth, mucous membranes, skeletal and soft tissues

VITAMIN C: for healthy gums and teeth, iron absorption and wound healing

CALCIUM: for building strong bones and teeth

IRON: for formation of hemoglobin (carries oxygen in blood) and myoglobin (carries oxygen in muscle)

Food labels are useful for comparing different foods and knowing what you're eating—but don't get too bogged down with specifics. Canada's Food Guide to Healthy Eating makes it easy to follow the recommendations that help you eat an overall balanced diet.

If a package is sold as one portion (such as yogurt or juice), the nutrition information usually applies to the whole package.

 Use the following simple tool to visualize how much fat or carbohydrates you're eating:

1 teaspoon oil = 5 grams fat
1 slice bread = 15 grams carbohydrates

The Canadian Food Inspection Agency is responsible for enforcing regulations and verifying industry compliance. At the time of writing there are still no labelling regulations related to food biotechnology, that is, genetically modified organisms (GMOs).

2. The ingredient list

The product's ingredients are listed here in *descending* order by quantity. At the top of the list is the ingredient that there's *most* of. At the bottom of the list is the ingredient there's *least* of. The list is especially useful if you are on a special diet, have food allergies or need to avoid a particular ingredient.

 Reading labels can help you get the most value for your money. If two similar products cost the same but one has more of the key ingredient, it might be a better choice. For instance, apple juice lists apple juice as the first ingredient. The first ingredients in apple drink are water and sugar.

How to speak label-ese

Here's a list of many of the different words for fat, sugar and salt that you'll find on labels.

Fats	ᴥ fat, lard, shortening
	ᴥ hydrogenated vegetable oils
	ᴥ vegetable oil
	ᴥ coconut/palm oils, tropical oils
	ᴥ mono and diglycerides, tallow
Sugars	ᴥ sugar, honey, molasses
	ᴥ dextrose, sucrose, fructose
	ᴥ maltose, lactose (words that end in -ose)
	ᴥ dextrin, maltodextrin, invert sugar
	ᴥ maple syrup, corn syrup, malt syrup
Salts	ᴥ salt, MSG
	ᴥ anything with the word sodium
	ᴥ baking soda, baking powder, brine
	ᴥ kelp, soy sauce

Read between the lines. If enriched white flour is the first ingredient on the list, that loaf of bread you're looking at is unlikely to be high in fibre. And if hydrogenated oil or shortening is at the top, those cookies you like are probably high in fat. Also remember that even though sugar may not head the list of ingredients, it may be there in quantity. Check the Nutrition Facts table for the bigger picture.

- "Fortified" or "enriched" means that nutrients are added or that some of the nutrients lost in processing have been restored. For instance, milk is enriched with vitamins A and D.
- "May contain" means an ingredient is optional.

Here are the Claims
3. Nutrient content claims

High fibre, low sodium, fat free. On packaging you often see words like these that highlight specific nutritional features of a food. Be reassured that it's not hype; the product meets certain criteria. The use of these words is strictly regulated by Health Canada so that they mean what they say. (See Appendix, Nutrient Content Claims, page 148.) Here's a primer to some of the more common claims:

"Free"

This nutrient or ingredient is contained in an amount so small that health experts consider it nutritionally insignificant. *Caution:* a "fat-free" product is not necessarily low in calories. It may contain sugar to boost the flavour. A "sugar-free" food means it is free of energy. The one exception is chewing gum.

"Low"

The food has a very small amount of the nutrient claimed. *Caution:* foods "low in saturated fat" or "cholesterol-free" must also be low in trans fats—since saturated fats, cholesterol and trans fats may increase the risk of heart disease—but they are not necessarily low in total fat. For example, vegetable oils contain no cholesterol but are still high in fat. Watching your total fat intake? The Nutrition Facts table tells you how much total fat the product contains.

"Reduced"

Compared with a similar "regular" product, this one contains at least 25% less of the nutrient. *Caution:* the amount of calories, fat, fibre, sugar, etc. could still be large, so be sure to check the Nutrition Facts table.

"High"

The food has a significant amount of the nutrient claimed.

"Light/Lite"

The product is reduced in calories or fat. *Caution:* the word "light" may also describe taste, colour or texture, as long as it is qualified. Read the label carefully to find out what part of the product is "light."

"No Added Sugar"

No sugars are added in processing or packaging. *Caution:* Although it may not have added sugar, a product could still be high in natural sugar. Watching your caloric intake? Check the Nutrition Facts table to find out how many calories one serving contains.

Nutrition claims highlight positive features of a product but they do not tell the whole story. Again, check the Nutrition Facts table for the bigger picture, and watch for the Health Check™ designation. It explains how that food is part of healthy eating.

4. Diet-related health claims

New to food labels in Canada are diet-related health claims. These messages reinforce the role of healthy eating as part of a lifestyle that can reduce the risk of developing a chronic disease, such as heart disease or cancer. Here are the claims that foods meeting Health Canada's nutritional criteria can make, if they are part of a healthy diet.

- A product *low in saturated fat and trans fats* may reduce the risk of heart disease.
- A food *rich in a variety of fruits and vegetables* may help reduce the risk of some types of cancer.
- A product *with adequate calcium and vitamin D* combined with regular physical activity helps to achieve strong bones and may reduce the risk of osteoporosis.
- A food *high in potassium and low in sodium* may reduce the risk of high blood pressure, a risk factor for stroke and heart disease.

Read on to find lots more tips on how to use labels wisely, as you load up your shopping cart the HeartSmart way.

Labels at a glance

- Remember to check the Nutrition Facts table and the ingredient list for an overview of what is in the food you buy.
- Read the nutrition claims to find out about the specific features of the food you eat.
- Let Health Check guide you to healthy food choices.

Careful shopping habits and storage smarts are among the most valuable skills you can acquire.

Gulp! Over 20 years a family of four is estimated to spend well over $100,000 in the supermarket. The good news is that the more you know, the better the food you can buy for your money. Careful shopping habits and storage smarts are among the most valuable skills you can acquire. Literally. Over time you can save thousands of dollars.

DID YOU KNOW? Food wasn't always trademarked. In great-grandmother's era all crackers came from the cracker barrel. If customers were dissatisfied the store owner simply bought from another source. Brand names came into being in the 1940s. This way the brand guaranteed quality and the same taste every time. But today no-name brands apply the same consistent quality control standards—and you're not paying the extra cents that subsidize advertising. Your decision.

Six cost-cutting tips

1. Store brands can save you a bundle. Often they are the least expensive, because they are not advertised like popular brand names. Is there a difference? Judge for yourself. Compare ingredient lists and read the Nutrition Facts tables if available. Ask your family or friends to taste both products (without telling them which is which) and let them decide.

2. Larger doesn't always mean cheaper. Don't always buy
    the biggest size. Compare the unit price of different
    sizes of similar items to see if you're really saving
    money. Check the little tab on the supermarket shelf
    which displays the price per gram or per millilitre. It's
    information worth looking at.

3. Buy in bulk...sometimes. Scooping out as much as
    you need from a bin may not be cheaper, especially if
    you need to buy large quantities. Sounds silly, doesn't
    it? But in fact, you get more value in "bulk" buying
    when you only need small quantities. Pre-packaged
    items are usually more economical for larger pur-
    chases. Look for the scales in this section of the
    supermarket and weigh the amount you buy so you
    won't be surprised when you get to the check-out.

    Buying warehouse-sized packages of cereal is a
    terrific idea if you have teenagers. You'll never run out
    and the price is considerably lower too. But that
    family-sized jar of fresh salsa will only be a super buy
    if you have space to store it and can use it up before
    the "best before" date.

4. Check local flyers for seasonal foods and weekly
    specials, but think twice about running around from
    one store to another to pick up your weekly purchases.
    Figure out how much time you'll spend. Gas costs too.

    Enjoy seasonal produce for all it's worth—and
    stash some in the freezer. That way you'll have home-
    frozen raspberries in the middle of winter for a lot
    less than the cost of the imported fresh ones.

5. Eat more vegetable proteins. Try peanut butter
    sandwiches, lentil soup with crackers, baked beans
    with corn bread or tofu with rice and stir-fried
    veggies. All offer high-quality nutrition at lower prices.

6. Take the extra time at home to store food wisely to
    ensure that it doesn't end up in the garbage can. The
    Penny Wise icon will point you to storage tips for each
    food group throughout the book.

Section *1* of your shopping cart

Grains

Vegetables and Fruit

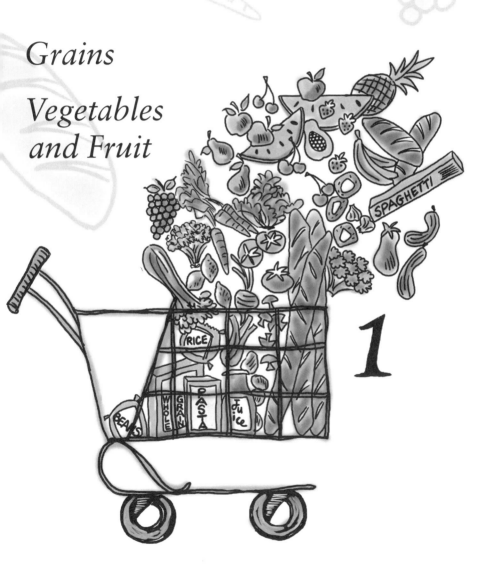

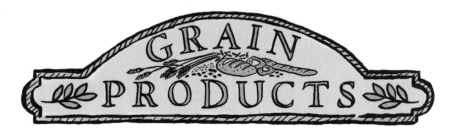

GRAIN PRODUCTS

Fill up the big #1 part of your shopping cart—load up on whole grains.

HeartSmart™ shoppers, we're on our way—but put on the brakes for a moment before we get going. Notice I said whole grains, not refined grains. Low in fat and loaded with fibre and nutrients, they're a terrific way to add variety to your diet. So feel free to fill the #1 part of your cart.

And what a wealth of choices you've got. Bakery shelves bulge with whole-wheat breads, buns, bagels, rolls and pitas. Whole-wheat pasta tempts with all its different shapes. Brown, wild, wehani…explore the world of rice. Check out the delicious "ancient" grains too, like bulgur, quinoa and cornmeal.

Grains are warming in winter and many make tasty main-dish salads. Add a handful of barley to a vegetable soup, and suddenly soup becomes supper. Making brown rice? Just add meat, poultry, fish or tofu and lots of cubed fresh vegetables (a great way to use leftovers) and you have a meal. And another nice piece of news: eaten in moderation, grains aren't only a great way to keep your health on track; they are easy on your fat budget. What's more, they're generally a bargain.

Eat more whole grains and you'll be doing your bit for the environment too. The same land required to raise beef for one person can grow enough rice to feed 24 people or wheat to feed 15.

Pile up the #1 part of your HeartSmart shopping cart with whole-grain products, and eat them more often.

Take five—and more if you can

Canada's Food Guide to Healthy Eating recommends 5–12 servings of grains a day. Hard to eat that much? Not a bit.

One serving means:
1 slice bread	3/4 cup (175 mL) hot cereal
1/2 bagel, pita or bun	1 ounce (30 g) cold cereal
1/2 cup (125 mL) pasta or rice (cooked)	

Fat budgeting with grain products

Most grains are low in fat. That's why it's so easy to load up the #1 part of your cart. Choose a variety of foods from the grain group to get many important nutrients.

Check the fat budget list and decide how you want to spend your fat budget.

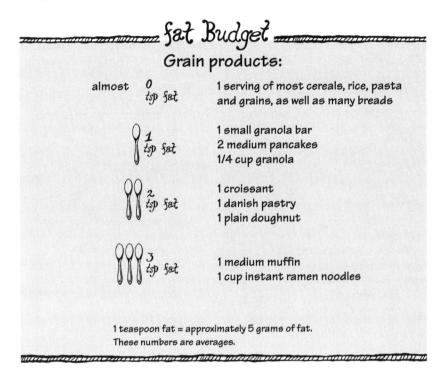

fat Budget

Grain products:

almost **0** *tsp fat*	1 serving of most cereals, rice, pasta and grains, as well as many breads
1 *tsp fat*	1 small granola bar 2 medium pancakes 1/4 cup granola
2 *tsp fat*	1 croissant 1 danish pastry 1 plain doughnut
3 *tsp fat*	1 medium muffin 1 cup instant ramen noodles

1 teaspoon fat = approximately 5 grams of fat.
These numbers are averages.

To find out what nutrients grain products offer and where they fit in the total nutrition picture, see Appendix, page 144.

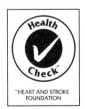

"HEART AND STROKE FOUNDATION

Look for grain products that are low-fat and a source of fibre.

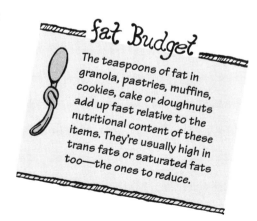

fat Budget

The teaspoons of fat in granola, pastries, muffins, cookies, cake or doughnuts add up fast relative to the nutritional content of these items. They're usually high in trans fats or saturated fats too—the ones to reduce.

Get fired up about fibre

The more fibre you eat, the easier it is for your intestinal tract to function smoothly. The easier it is to maintain a healthy weight too. Eating carbohydrates helps you cut back on calorie-dense fats and sweets. Research shows that fibre may help to prevent certain forms of cancer and lower our cholesterol. We used to think fibre was useless. Big mistake. Now we know just how important it really is.

Fibre is a type of carbohydrate found only in plants. It's a special component of food that isn't absorbed. Instead, it passes right through your system. There are two types—soluble and insoluble.

Soluble fibre can help control blood sugar. It can also help lower blood cholesterol, especially if it is high.

Insoluble fibre helps to prevent and control bowel problems and may be important in the prevention of certain cancers.

You'll find soluble fibre in:

- Oat bran
- Oatmeal
- Legumes (dried beans, peas and lentils)
- Pectin-rich fruits (apples, strawberries, citrus fruits, pears)

You'll find insoluble fibre in:

- Wheat bran and wheat-bran cereals
- Whole-grain foods like whole-wheat bread
- Fruit and vegetables, including skins and seeds when practical

Double your fibre! The typical North American diet contains about 12–15 grams of dietary fibre. Most authorities recommend aiming for 25–35 grams. Here's how:

- Fibre-rich cereal for breakfast
- Raisins, banana or orange slices on your cereal
- Low-fat bran or oatmeal muffin
- Whole-grain breads
- Tons of veggies and fruit for snacks
- Beans, peas and lentils
- High-fibre cereal on casseroles

ALL STAR TIP

Suddenly increasing your fibre may leave you feeling bloated. Up your fibre intake gradually and be sure to drink up to 8 cups (2 litres) of fluid daily (see page 16).

Many products contain fibre—but how much? Reading the fine print will tell you.

If the package says:	It means this much fibre per serving:
"Source of dietary fibre"	at least 2 grams
"High source of dietary fibre"	at least 4 grams
"Very high source of dietary fibre"	at least 6 grams

A trip down the bakery aisle

Bagels, baguettes, French and Italian peasant breads, pita, pumpernickel, rye bread, English muffins, tortillas…can you believe the number of breads we have available? Bread can be a powerhouse of nutrition. It supplies a large part of our daily carbohydrate intake. It's also a good source of fibre, thiamin, riboflavin, niacin, iron and trace minerals. Just be sure you buy whole-grain whenever possible. Read the label before you buy. That way you'll know you're getting valuable fibre and nutrients.

Watching your weight? It used to be that a slice of bread contained roughly 80 calories. Today manufacturers produce breads that can be up to 130 calories per slice. If bread is a staple in your diet, check the Nutrition Facts table for the bread highest in fibre and lowest in calories. Look for bread with at least 2 to 3 grams of fibre per slice. Check the serving size. Is it for one or two slices?

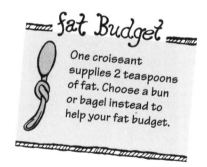

fat Budget

One croissant supplies 2 teaspoons of fat. Choose a bun or bagel instead to help your fat budget.

Is today's bread better bred? Not necessarily.

Great-grandmother had no choice. She had to serve bread made from stone-ground flour. Little did she know how healthy it was. Back then, only the inedible husk was removed when the miller ground the flour. As the wheat was ground between two stones, the husks were sifted or blown out. What was left was packed with nutrients. Along came modern times—and machinery that could get rid of not only the husk but also nutrient-rich wheat germ and high-fibre bran. All that was left was the smooth, white endosperm. White bread became a status symbol. Crunchy brown bread made from nutritious whole-grain flour was considered old-fashioned.

Then problems developed. Many people began to develop deficiencies of iron and the B vitamins niacin, thiamin and riboflavin. An Enrichment Act was passed in 1942 stating that these four nutrients must be added back to refined flour. This law is still in effect and so, whatever their colour, grain products, breads and cereals manufactured in Canada have been enriched with at least these four nutrients. Folate is now being added too.

But it's still not as nutritious as the original wheat grain. Many of the nutrients found in the whole grain—magnesium, zinc, vitamin B6, vitamin E, chromium and fibre—are lost in white bread.

Bread buying made easy

Boosting your fibre intake is easy if you get into the habit of buying whole-grain bread. Two slices (about 50 grams) can give you a mighty 4–6 grams of fibre or more. Since you're aiming for 25–35 grams a day, you can get a significant amount from the bread you eat.

For nutritious higher-fibre bread, look for the words "whole grain" or "stone ground" first on the ingredient list. Wheat bran also boosts the fibre content. Don't be misled: the words "wheat flour," "wheat bread" or "cracked wheat" on the wrapper mean only that the bread is made from flour that comes from wheat. Similarly, if a label says a bread contains 100% whole-wheat flour, it may not mean that 100% of it is whole-wheat. Many breads are made with more than one flour. Check the ingredient list to see what other flours are listed and where the whole wheat is found on the list. Remember, the first ingredient on the list is present in the greatest quantity.

Label Smarts If a bread is labelled "no cholesterol," ignore this claim. Most breads don't contain cholesterol anyway. Cholesterol comes from animal foods.

All Star Tip Soft corn or flour tortillas make a great base for tacos, salads or Mexican pizza. All contain less fat than the crispy kind.

Penny Wise Help buns and bread keep their freshness when you're buying them from bulk bins. Store crusty ones in paper bags and soft ones in plastic bags.

Q&A *Does dark coloured bread mean that it's high in fibre?* Unfortunately, colour isn't a reliable clue. Bread can be made with refined flour and the dough darkened with molasses, caramel or cocoa. Taking a good look at the label will help.

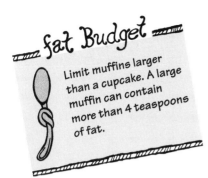

Fat Budget

Limit muffins larger than a cupcake. A large muffin can contain more than 4 teaspoons of fat.

DID YOU KNOW?

Muffin mania began in the 1970s when the news about fibre first came to the fore. Bran, fibre...it all sounded so healthy. In fact, most muffins contain relatively little bran (and some none at all). More to the point, many can be loaded with fat and calories.

What about pancake mixes?

For many people it's a weekend tradition—and mixes make it so easy. Pancakes are an OK option; they contain very little fat. But watch the amount that's added at the table. Two tips work in my house: one, be more generous with the syrup than the spread. It has half the calories. Two, switch to a non-hydrogenated, low-fat margarine. It's easier to spread so you use less.

HeartSmart Tip

Check your favourite cookbook for a classic pancake recipe, then make some HeartSmart switches:
ﻉ Egg whites—two for each whole egg ﻉ Lower-fat milk instead of whole milk ﻉ Whole-wheat flour instead of white ﻉ Add wheat bran and wheat germ to increase the fibre ﻉ Reduce the oil ﻉ Cook in a nonstick pan

Banana breads and zucchini loaves sound wonderfully healthy. Are they?

We picture fresh fruits and vegetables when we hear their names. Vitamin rich. Fibre galore. Unfortunately, the rest of the ingredients are often the same as those in regular cake. Very little fruit or vegetable may be used. Try a homemade, lower-fat variety instead.

ALL-STAR TIP

• Add wheat germ to up the nutritional value of all-purpose refined flour. Use whole-grain flour whenever possible.

• To make your own self-rising flour, add 1 tablespoon (15 mL) baking powder and 1/4 teaspoon (1 mL) salt to 3 cups (750 mL) flour.

The serious shopper's guide to cereals

Cereal can be the foundation of a fast, nutritious breakfast. Ready-to-eat cereal with lower-fat milk is a good snack for kids of all ages, but it can also provide an overload of added sugar and fat. Fortunately, the label tells all. Choose wisely. A good rule of thumb? The shorter the ingredient list the better.

So what's a typical serving size?

A typical serving size is:
1/3 cup (80 mL) bran cereal, concentrated;
1/2 cup (125 mL) bran cereal, flaked;
2/3 cup (175 mL) other ready-to-eat, unsweetened cereals;
1 1/2 cups (375 mL) puffed cereal; and
1/2 cup (125 mL) cooked cereal.

If you eat more than that amount, adjust the values on the labels accordingly.

Looking for more fibre?

Choose a cereal that has at least 2 grams of fibre per serving. The fibre will be listed under carbohydrate content. Cereal is a great way to increase your daily fibre intake. A high-fibre cereal has 4 grams of fibre per serving, and you can obtain as much as 13 grams per serving from some all-bran varieties. Granolas may have less fibre than you think. When whole grain is the first ingredient, it's present in the greatest quantity.

Cutting back on fat?

Most cereals are low in fat since they are based on grains, which contain little fat. Ideally they should contain no more than 1 to 3 grams of fat per serving. Granolas may have 5 grams or more, and the fat is often highly saturated coconut or palm oil, or partly saturated hydrogenated vegetable oil. Nuts and seeds add to the fat content. Check the label and look for lower-fat varieties. Remember that nuts and seeds add healthy fats.

Looking for added vitamins and minerals?

Cereal is typically fortified with 10% to 25% of some of the daily vitamins and minerals we require. A great idea, because cereal is the way that many of us start every day. But do you need the "new and improved" cereals that claim to be fortified with 100% of the vitamins and minerals? Not really. Cereal is not all you will be eating during the day. You will get vitamins and minerals from many other food sources. The milk you add will also contain added minerals and vitamins.

Are cereals that contain oats a wild idea?

In fact, they're a good one. Oat bran may reduce blood cholesterol levels. It contains soluble fibre. You have to consume a lot to make a significant difference—about six servings of oats daily, but every bit helps. Try oats in many forms. Old-fashioned rolled oats, quick-cooking rolled oats and instant oats all have similar nutritional value.

Instant oatmeal retains most of the nutrient value of whole and rolled oats, but usually has salt and sugar added to it.

Commercial brands of granola and muesli can be high in fat (granola usually more so than muesli). They're often high in tropical oils and include added ingredients such as coconut, nuts and seeds. Read the label and choose the newer low-fat options.

Try sprinkling fibre on your cereal

- WHEAT BRAN is the outer shell of the wheat kernel. It is the most concentrated form of insoluble fibre there is. Go slowly. Adding too much too fast can affect your body's absorption of calcium and iron, and cause gas and bloating. Allow your body to adapt by increasing your wheat bran intake gradually.

- WHEAT GERM is the embryo of the wheat kernel. It's high in polyunsaturated fat and vitamin E and B vitamins. Store in the fridge so it won't go rancid. Defatted wheat germ (it contains less vitamin E) can be kept in your cupboard.

Psyllium is the seed of the plantain plant. It is a natural fibre that may help lower blood cholesterol and keep bowels regular. Check for this ingredient in your high-fibre cereal.

Pasta—use your noodles...but wisely

Convenience? You can't beat it. Twelve minutes in the pot for dry pasta and you can have a bountiful bowl on the table. It's delicious. It's versatile. It's no wonder it shows up on so many tables. But slow down. Eating oodles of noodles made from refined flour is not a great idea—especially if you are trying to manage your weight. One cup of pasta is equal to two servings of grains. How many cups do you normally have?

A healthier idea is to choose a smaller serving of whole-wheat pasta and load up your sauce with veggies and a lower-fat protein (see Mighty Meals, Pasta Power, page 137).

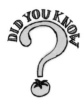

Pasta may have been the very first convenience food. Three thousand years ago, the Greeks and Romans discovered how to make pastas out of water and ground grain, which they could dry and take with them on long journeys.

- Pastas called "noodles" contain some egg solids—some cholesterol but not enough to concern yourself about if you rarely choose them.

- Asian noodles are sometimes called imitation noodles because they are not made with egg. They include bean thread noodles, buckwheat noodles (soba), "egg" noodles, rice noodles and wheat noodles.

- Most pasta is made from wheat. If you are allergic to wheat, look for pasta made with other grains.

The instant appeal of instant noodles

I'll admit, oriental instant noodles (e.g., Japanese ramen) are quick, tasty, made in a minute. Precooked and then dried, they are packaged with a packet of seasonings. All you have to do is add boiling water. Yes, they're simple but be careful; they're not that nutritious. These noodles are usually deep-fried in highly saturated fat such as lard or palm oil, and they are high in salt.

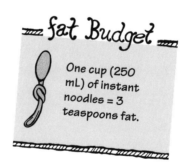

Fat Budget

One cup (250 mL) of instant noodles = 3 teaspoons fat.

Choose whole-wheat pasta and double your fibre intake from 2 to 4 grams per cup.

Try "new kinds" of noodles

- High-protein pasta made with soy flour
- Whole-wheat pasta high in fibre and minerals
- No-yolk egg noodles

What are most pastas made from?

The hard spring wheat called durum is unsuitable for breads and cakes but ideal for pasta. The durum wheat is refined and ground into a white flour called semolina. When mixed with water and made into a dough, it can be cut into a vast range of shapes and sizes. Semolina has more protein, vitamins and minerals than ordinary all-purpose flour. It cooks up firm and slightly chewy, or as they say in Italy, *al dente.*

Is fresh pasta a better choice than dried pasta?

Not necessarily. Fresh pasta contains more water, so you get less, kilo for kilo, for your money. Dried pasta can be stored for a long time without any nutrient loss. Cooked or fresh pasta can be frozen for later use.

What gives pasta its different colours and textures?

Often vegetables—beets, carrots or spinach—are used to add colour. Be careful: these are such small amounts that coloured pastas are no more nutritious than white ones. Seasoning such as chili peppers or lemon can add another dimension to pasta. Whole-wheat pastas have a different texture and taste (they need longer cooking) but they do contain more fibre, vitamins and minerals and have a slightly higher protein content.

How can I find a sauce that's low in fat?

Many tomato-based sauces are low in fat, but not all. Check the Nutrition Facts table or read the ingredients. If cream, cheese, meats or fats are listed near the top of the list, find another sauce.

What are good ways to boost your pasta sauces?

Not by adding cream, butter or cheese—which means limit that Fettuccini Alfredo! Use a tomato sauce as a base, and add tuna or scallops, or make a luscious and authentically Italian primavera sauce with tomatoes, fresh vegetables steamed briefly and a touch of white wine. Delicious.

fun food...fast

Momma Ramona's fresh tomato sauce

This is a cinch to make and it explodes with flavour. Serves four.

2 tsp (10 mL) olive oil—or use stock
2 cloves garlic, finely chopped
1 1/2 lb (750 g) chopped firm roma tomatoes or a 28-oz (796 g) can
   tomatoes
big pinch basil, parsley, oregano and rosemary
salt and pepper to taste
1 tbsp (15 mL) parmesan cheese

Heat oil in nonstick frying pan. Sauté garlic until lightly browned. Add tomatoes and, if using fresh, cook until tomatoes release some juice. Break up tomatoes with a wooden spoon. Stir in herbs (use at least double for fresh herbs) and cook for about 5 minutes, until sauce reduces. Season to taste. Serve immediately over cooked pasta. Sprinkle with cheese. One tablespoon of grated parmesan cheese provides less than 1/2 tsp fat and just 25 calories. Or try the new lower-fat parmesan cheese. Enjoy!

Cooking rice and other grains

Rice is *really* nice nutritionally. When we were growing up, most of us viewed rice as an extra—the little white mound on the side of the plate. Yet half the world eats rice as its staple food. Chinese tradition has it that a person who has not eaten rice has not fully eaten.

Rice is easy to cook. Measure it first, allowing about 1/3 cup (75 mL) per person. Rinse thoroughly until water runs clear. Place in a pot and add twice the amount of water or add flavour by using broth or juice instead of water. Bring to a boil, stir well, cover and reduce heat. Simmer for 20 minutes, or longer if it's a higher-fibre rice (see Quick Guide to Cooking Grains, page 54). Fluff rice with a fork before serving so that the steam can escape and the grains don't stick together.

If you cannot serve rice immediately, cover with a tea towel and place the lid back on—this will prevent rice turning gummy.

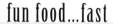
fun food...fast
Quick and nippy rice recipes

Rice Pilaf

Sauté 1 chopped onion in 1 tbsp (15 mL) of hot stock. Add 1 cup (250 mL) rice and cook two minutes, or until rice becomes opaque. Add 2 cups (500 mL) boiling stock. Cover and cook until liquid is absorbed. Season with cinnamon and ginger. Toss with a scant handful of chopped nuts or dried fruit.

Vegetable Paella

Sauté 1 chopped onion, a chopped garlic clove and 1 cup (250 mL) uncooked rice in 2 tbsp (30 mL) hot stock until onions are transparent and rice lightly browned. Add 1 1/2 cups (375 mL) boiling stock, 1 cup (250 mL) stewed tomatoes with juice, and a pinch of paprika, cayenne pepper and crushed saffron. Bring to boil, reduce heat and simmer 10 minutes. Add a chopped-up pepper, 1/2 cup (125 mL) each of frozen peas and corn niblets. Cover and simmer again for 10 minutes until liquid is absorbed and rice is tender.

Green Rice

Add freshly chopped parsley or cilantro to cooked rice. Experiment with other herbs.

Main Meal Rice

Simply mix cut-up cooked vegetables, lean meat, chicken, fish or legumes with cooked rice. A great way to stretch leftovers.

White rice, brown rice. Short grain, long grain. Red rice, wild rice. What a fabulous way to add variety to the foods we eat.

White rice makes up nearly 99% of the rice we eat. Too bad. Even in Asia, nearly all the rice eaten is polished, which strips it of fibre, protein, vitamins and minerals.

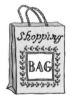

Whole-grain rice is rich in phytochemicals. Create your own wild grain mix with a medley of colours: brown whole-grain rice, black japonica, red wehani and brown jasmine.

Different shapes of rice give different results when you cook them. The shorter the grain, the stickier the rice. Long grains are ideal for casseroles and stuffing.

Q&A *What's the scoop on brown rice?*
Choose good and chewy brown or whole-grain rice and you're getting the whole unpolished rice grain. Only the husk and a little of the bran is removed. Though it takes a bit longer to cook than white rice, it contains more fibre and minerals. Unlike other rice, it's also a source of vitamin E.

HeartSmart Tip

How much fibre in a cup of cooked rice?

1 cup	Fibre
White rice	1 g
Brown rice	3 g
Wild rice	4 g

Choose brown rice over white rice and increase your fibre intake from 1 gram to 3 grams per cup.

What's the word on parboiled or converted rice?
The word is yes! This rice goes through a special steam-pressure process which pushes some of its nutrients into the starchy centre of each grain so that vitamins are not lost when the rice is milled. Unfortunately it is lower in fibre than brown rice. The word "parboiled" might lead you to think that this kind of rice cooks quickly. In fact, it takes just as long to cook as ordinary rice.

Any thoughts on precooked or instant rice?
These are the most highly processed and expensive rices. Even when enriched, they offer the least nourishment.

Fat Budget

If you use a packaged rice mix, you don't need to add fat even though the box says to. The rice tastes fine without it—and that would help your fat budget. It is also just as simple to make your own seasoned rice from scratch using your favourite herbs.

Grains galore

It's time to spread the word. The best-kept secret around is all the deliciously different grains you'll find in your supermarket. Popular staples of Middle Eastern and Mediterranean cuisine, most of them cook in a flash—often faster than rice or pasta.

Amaranth
An ancient Aztec grain. The only grain that supplies a good amount of calcium. Good source of iron too. Each kernel is as tiny as a poppy seed. Most appetizing when added to another grain. Cook in broth or juice and combine with stir-fries.

Barley
Delicious in soups (see recipe on page 138), stews and casseroles, and as a cereal. Whole (Scotch) barley is more nutritious than the polished (pearl) barley and takes longer to cook.

Buckwheat
This is actually a seed. Whole, it's called groats. Roasted and hulled, it's known as kasha. Before cooking, add beaten egg to coat the grains—this will prevent the grains from sticking together. To cut the added fat, use beaten egg whites.

Quinoa
Pronounced "keen-wa," this is a light, non-sticky grain with a delicate flavour. Substitute for rice or use as a base for salads. It is called the mother grain because it has more complete protein than any other grain and is high in vitamins and minerals. Not as expensive as it may seem because it increases 3 to 4 times during cooking. It's cooked when grains are translucent and turn into spirals.

Cornmeal
Ground corn kernels. Make Italian polenta by bringing 3 cups of lightly salted water or stock to a boil, then slowly pour in 1 cup of cornmeal (to prevent lumps, add a little water to the cornmeal first, blend and then add). Stir constantly until mixture starts to come away from the sides of the pan. Can be pressed in pan, cut into squares and broiled.

Wheat
Wheat berries—the whole-wheat kernels are high in nutrition. Enjoy as a cereal or add to breads and muffins. Keep in the fridge because the whole grain contains natural oils which can turn rancid.
Bulgur—or cracked wheat, often called the rice of the Middle East. Can be served in many innovative ways—as a main event, side dish or cold salad.
Couscous—a North African specialty, couscous is made from semolina and is actually a form of pasta. Add to boiling water, turn heat off and leave to cook.

Quick guide to cooking grains (check package for instructions)

GRAINS (1 CUP)	WATER	TIME (MINUTES)
Amaranth	1 cup (250 mL)	30
Barley		
Scotch (whole)	4 cups (1 L)	100
Pearl (polished)	3 cups (750 mL)	55
Buckwheat		
Groats (whole)	2 cups (500 mL)	15
Kasha (roasted, hulled)	5 cups (1.25 L)	12
Millet	3 cups (750 mL)	30
Oats		
Whole	2 cups (500 mL)	60
Rolled	2 cups (500 mL)	10
Quinoa	2 cups (500 mL)	15
Rice		
Long grain	2 cups (500 mL)	20 or longer
Short grain	2 cups (500 mL)	20 or longer
White basmati	1 1/2 cups (375 mL)	15
Wild rice	4 cups (1 L)	50
Wheat		
Wheat berries	3 cups (750 mL)	60
Bulgur	2 cups (500 mL)	15
Couscous	2 cups (500 mL)	15

fun food...fast
Great grain boosters

- To boost flavour, cook grains in broth or diluted orange or tomato juice.
- For an Asian twist, season with soy sauce, ground sesame seeds and grated ginger. Or try curry powder with chopped cilantro, peppers, green onion and orange slices. For a Mediterranean flavour, add oregano, basil, marjoram and chopped parsley.
- For a tasty hot meal or side dish, toss cooked grains with cooked vegetables (e.g., carrots, celery, mushrooms), fresh herbs and your favourite low-fat dressing.
- For delicious cold salads, add cold cooked grains to tuna, chopped vegetables (e.g., peas, mushrooms, peppers, green onions) and toss with a vinaigrette dressing or lemon juice and a dash of olive oil.
- For tasty thickened soups, add grains to stock pot.
- To get used to the nutty flavour of many of these grains, combine them with milder grains—add brown rice to kasha (roasted buckwheat).

The bran and germ layers of whole wheat are rich in phytochemicals that may help to reduce the risk of cancer and heart disease. Whole grains preserve these substances—so toss those wheat berries, cracked wheat, bulgur and other high-fibre grains into the #1 part of your shopping cart.

Cookies? Pastries?

OK, the truth. No way can you justify cookies and pastries from a nutritional standpoint—they're usually made from refined flour and loaded with fat and calories. But who eats them for nutrition anyway? In fact, statistics reveal that each of us eats about 5 kilograms of cookies a year! Balance your cookie craving by keeping a close eye on the other fats you eat that day. That way you'll still have your fat budget under control.

Cookies contain flour, fat and sugar. Your best bets are those that are high in whole-wheat flour and low in fat and calories.

We may be getting older, but our diet may not be getting better. Research shows that today women eat more unhealthy trans fats in the form of baked goods than before.

Some cookie facts

No matter what fat is used, the less the better. Fat-free cookies may still be loaded with sugar. Read the label, and check the calories per serving.

• A cookie that is "calorie reduced" means that it has fewer calories than the original product—but it doesn't necessarily mean that it's low in calories. Once again, let the label be your guide and compare with other choices.

• "Whole-grain" on granola bars means they may contain a small quantity of oats, but the amount may be insignificant relative to the added fat and calories.

Made with oats, nuts and seeds, granola bars are high in protein and fibre. They may seem to be a wise choice but in fact they are usually high in fat and calories too—often boosted by other ingredients such as miniature marshmallows, or chocolate or caramel chips. Check the label to learn the fat and calories in a serving size. Enjoy them if you want, but keep your fat budget in mind—and choose the new products lower in fat and calories.

Some of the wisest choices in the cookie aisle are some of the oldest ones. Gingersnaps and graham crackers are both low in fat. So are fruit bars, plain wafers and animal crackers. The good news…manufacturers know we can't resist the cookie jar so they're hard at work inventing cookies that are lower in fat and calories. Keep your eyes open.

Putting the crunch on crackers

Crackers can be a wise choice if you're watching your calorie, fat and fibre intake. But how do you know which to pick?

- Look for as little fat and salt as possible.
- Choose crackers made from whole-grain flour whenever you can.
- Read the ingredients and make sure that whole-wheat flour is top of the list.

Big crackers, small crackers, ones you can eat by the handful, ones that take several bites—no wonder a serving size of crackers is anybody's guess. Only you know how many you eat at a time. Try to get the most crackers and most fibre you can for the fewest calories.

Cracker countdown

These are all low-fat choices:

If a cracker is greasy to the touch or leaves a greasy mark on paper, it's high in fat.

- Flatbreads and crispbreads
- Water crackers
- Rice cakes
- Melba toasts
- Matzos

Choose those with the most fibre.

Grains at a glance

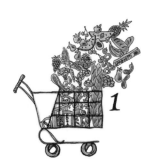

1. Look for whole-grain products.
2. Choose cereals with at least 2 grams fibre per serving. More is better.
3. Experiment with varieties of grains.

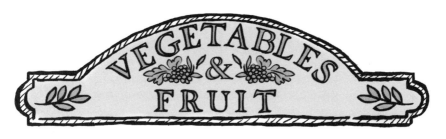

VEGETABLES & FRUIT

Feel free to fill the big #1 part of your cart, loading it up with veggies and fruit

Hope you left lots of space in the large #1 part of your shopping cart, because here's where HeartSmart™ shoppers can really go crazy. Run riot! Fill your cart to the top. Along with grain products, vegetables and fruit should form the bulk of your diet.

We all grew up being told to eat our vegetables and somewhere along the line, we got the idea that they weren't delicious. A crispy green salad? Sweet little peas just out of the pod? A snappy handful of carrot sticks? Tiny new potatoes? *Not delicious?!!*

Vegetables can be b-o-o-oring if you serve the same ones day after day, especially at the end of the season. So try some new faces. From blue potatoes to yellow tomatoes, your supermarket is brimming with different varieties. Try scarlet kale or chopped red cabbage to jazz up a plain green salad. Add colour to mashed potatoes with a handful of parsley—vibrant green and available year round. Zip up a fish dish with jalapeno peppers. Even a little makes a huge difference.

And think about fruit. Bite into a juicy sun-warmed peach. Chill out with cold cubes of honeydew on a hot summer day. Picture the sharp yellows and greens of lemons and limes piled in a wicker basket. Wander the world of tropical fruit. Try chunks of papaya on your breakfast cereal (and use the seeds in salad dressing, see page 76). Serve yellow-orange slices of gorgeous mango for dessert. Snack on a bowl of lychees when they're in season.

No wonder supermarkets display their produce with pride. In fact, it's the only section so beautiful that it often gets to look at itself in a mirror. We often judge where we shop by how fresh and attractive its produce looks. Fruits and vegetables are loaded with nutrients. Antioxidants, phytochemicals, complex carbohydrates, fibre—they're full of the substances that we can feel free to eat in abundance. And oh, so low in fat.

Want some proof? Hundreds of studies now confirm that plant foods play a special role in the prevention of heart disease, obesity and cancer.

Take five! And more if you can

Canada's Food Guide to Healthy Eating recommends 5–10 servings a day from the produce section. If that sounds like a lot, relax, it isn't.

One serving means:
1 medium fruit or vegetable	1/2 cup (125 mL) fruit juice
1/2 cup (125 mL) cooked vegetables	1 cup salad

1 serving fruit or vegetable = the size of a tennis ball

Here's how 10 servings might work for you and your family on a typical day.

Breakfast: a small glass of orange juice or half a grapefruit

Mid-morning: an apple

Lunch: minestrone soup or a large salad, plus lettuce and tomato in your sandwich

Supper: soup or salad plus 1 or 2 cups of vegetables, fresh grapes or a half cantaloupe for dessert

Snack: frozen berries or a banana

Fat budgeting with vegetables and fruits

Most vegetables and fruits are low in fat. That's why it's so easy to load up the #1 part of your cart. Choose a variety to get a range of important nutrients.

Check the fat budget list and decide how you want to spend your fat budget.

Fat Budget
Vegetables and fruits:

0 tsp fat	most vegetables and fruits
	fruit and vegetable juices

1 tsp fat

2 tbsp (30 mL) shredded coconut
7 olives*

2 tsp fat

1/2 cup (125 mL) hash browns
10 french fries

3 tsp fat

1/2 medium avocado*

1 teaspoon fat = approximately 5 grams of fat.
These numbers are averages.
* Budget your fat wisely. Choose these healthier fats more often.

To find out what nutrients vegetables and fruit offer and where they fit in the total nutrition picture, see Appendix, page 144.

fat Budget

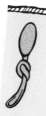

- What about fruit pies? Too high in fat to be considered a fruit serving. Sorry.
- Go slow with french fries. Made from potatoes, yes, but the added fat can burden your fat budget.
- The fat in olives and avocados is mostly monounsaturated — a wise way to spend your fat budget.

"A palette for your palate" is the ideal way to balance your fruit and vegetables. Fill your cart with as many different colours as you can. GREEN lettuce, broccoli, peas, green beans and zucchini. YELLOW squash, grapefruit and bananas. RED sweet peppers, tomatoes and apples. ORANGE squash and apricots. A wide spectrum of colours means you're getting the full spectrum of nutrients and phyto-chemicals that fruit and vegetables offer. A bonus—on a plate, all those hues look extra appealing.

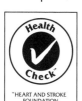

Look for fresh, frozen or canned vegetables or fruit, and REAL juice.

Extra! Extra! Read all about them

Fruits and vegetables come in their own gorgeous packaging but if they were sold like other products, imagine what it might say on their labels:

- *High in Fibre!*
- *No Cholesterol!*
- *Low Fat!*
- *With Phytochemicals and Antioxidants!*

What a bonanza. Fruit and vegetables are loaded with nutrients and low in calories. Nice to know if you want to stay healthy and manage your weight.

Eating a diet that contains a healthy amount of fibre may lessen your risk of developing heart disease, constipation, cancer of the colon, rectal cancer, breast cancer, obesity and diverticulosis.

An apple a day? Yes!

Look for this health claim on packaged foods containing fruits or vegetables: "A healthy diet rich in a variety of fruits and vegetables may help reduce the risk of some types of cancer."

Phytochemicals—the super nutrients

Pronounced "fight-o-chemicals," these nutrients are naturally present in plants, where they fight the stresses of harsh climate and infections. They also repel insects and protect plants from solar radiation.

Talk about hard-working multi-taskers! Although scientists are still trying to unlock the secrets of these nutrients, it seems phytochemicals may protect humans too, against conditions ranging from cancer to heart disease. Most appear to act as antioxidants (see page 61), protecting our cells from damage caused by exposure to smoke, air pollution and too much sunlight.

Phytochemicals flavour, colour or give foods their smell. One group, the polyphenols, includes flavonoids which add flavour to, for instance, garlic, shallots and onions. Carotenoids add colour to red peppers, blueberries, tomatoes and carrots.

Remember that phytochemicals and other healthful nutrients that occur naturally work together in the body in ways that scientists are only beginning to understand. So be wary of nutritional supplements; their dosages are not known and they have not been proven effective or safe. Load up instead with veggies and fruit.

 Can't remember the name of a particular phytochemical? You're not alone. Scientists have identified 4,000 phytochemicals so far and have studied only a few hundred.

You'll find phytochemicals in:

- 🐛 Cruciferous vegetables such as broccoli, cauliflower and cabbage
- 🐛 Legumes, especially soy products
- 🐛 Flaxseeds
- 🐛 Carrots, parsley, parsnips, turnips, citrus fruits
- 🐛 Garlic, onions, chives

Arm yourself with antioxidants

A rusting iron pipe and a cut apple that turns brown are both examples of what oxygen (oxidation) does in the wrong place at the wrong time. Oxidation can cause similar damage in our bodies.

Until a few years ago, we had not even heard of antioxidants. Now they're often in the headlines. Basically, antioxidants are chemical substances that help protect the body from oxygen's "bad side." By mopping up free radicals, they help to safeguard body cells. They may help prevent chronic disease such as heart disease and cancer, and premature aging.

Research suggests that four key antioxidants may come to the rescue: vitamins C and A (in the form of beta carotene) are plentiful in fruits and vegetables; vitamin E and the mineral selenium are the other two.

You'll find vitamin C in:

- 🐛 Vegetables: peppers, cauliflower, broccoli, brussels sprouts, sweet potatoes and snow peas
- 🐛 Fruit: citrus fruits, strawberries, papaya, melon and kiwis
- 🐛 Juice from these fruits or juice enriched with vitamin C

You'll find beta carotene in:

- 🐛 Dark green leafy vegetables such as collard greens, spinach, mustard greens, kale, broccoli and Swiss chard
- 🐛 Yellow and orange vegetables such as carrots, squash, pumpkins and sweet potatoes
- 🐛 Yellow and orange fruits such as melons, apricots, mangoes, papaya and peaches

Don't be fooled by beta carotene look-alikes. Sweet corn and beets may be the right colour but their colour doesn't come from beta carotene. Still good choices, but not for beta carotene.

Popeye was right. Spinach equals power—nutritional power. The amount of beta carotene in leafy green veggies seems to be linked to chlorophyll, the green pigment produced by photosynthesis. So, the darker the better. To up your antioxidant intake, choose deep orange or dark green vegetables and fruit at least every other day. Eating foods brilliant in "traffic-light colours" is definitely a "go."

The antioxidants vitamin E and selenium are not found in fruit or vegetables.

You'll find vitamin E in:

- foods that contain unsaturated fat, such as vegetable oils (except olive oil), wheat germ, peanut butter, nuts and seeds, and avocados.

You'll find selenium in:

- many foods, including Brazil nuts, meats, poultry, fish and grain products.

Fill up with folate or folic acid

Folate (a form of vitamin B found in foods) or folic acid (a synthetic version added to vitamin pills and some foods) may help protect against heart disease. Here's how. When your body metabolizes protein, it produces an amino acid called homocysteine, which breaks down into harmless substances with the help of folate and vitamins B6 and B12. Sometimes, due to a genetic or environmental defect, it accumulates instead. The result? It may damage the lining of the arteries and increase the risk of heart disease.

Experts recommend you get up to 400 mcg of folic acid or folate a day. Many multivitamins contain this amount. Load up on legumes, green leafy vegetables and fruit. Remember, folic acid or folate comes from the word "foliage."

You'll find folic acid in:

- Excellent sources: Lentils, chickpeas, kidney beans, asparagus, romaine lettuce, chicory greens, orange juice, pineapple juice, sunflower seeds.
- Good sources: Lima beans, corn, bean sprouts, broccoli, green peas, Brussels sprouts, beets, oranges, honeydew melon, raspberries, blackberries, avocados, roasted peanuts, wheat germ.

Grain products are now fortified with folic acid in both Canada and the United States.

To-mah-to or to-may-to—either way, should we say it often?

Tomatoes appear to be especially high in lycopene, an antioxidant that may help prevent cancer, especially prostate cancer, as well as heart disease. Processed or cooked tomatoes are a better choice than raw tomatoes. Heat breaks down the cell walls of the tomato, freeing the lycopene that would normally pass through your digestive system. So, try tomato juice, pasta sauce or pizza sauce, tomato purée, tomato sauce or tomato soup.

Watch the sodium content of processed products if you have high blood pressure. Tomato paste tends to have less than tomato sauce or canned tomatoes.

How about frozen fruit?

Feel free to buy it. Picked and chilled at its prime, frozen fruit has the same nutrients as fresh. The trip from orchard to freezer often takes only a few hours. Frozen fruits are processed without cooking and so there is little if any nutrient loss. Give those frozen raspberries a shake before they go in your cart. A rattling sound means they haven't thawed, then refrozen. And remember to check the label—sometimes sugar is added, which boosts the calories.

What about canned fruit and vegetables?

An easy, penny-wise way to add colour to your plate, canned fruits and veggies are super convenient—and they offer variety year round. Canned products today retain much of their vitamins and minerals, though water-soluble vitamins run the risk of being destroyed by the high temperatures called for in the canning process. To preserve minerals such as calcium or iron that may leach into the canning liquid, add the liquid to soups. Or use it instead of water when you put the rice pot on. Remember, canned vegetables are often heavily salted. Look for "low salt" on the label. Canned fruits may be packed in syrup which can boost the calorie content. Choose water-packed or juice-packed instead. Use the Nutrition Facts table to compare calories.

Should I add dried fruit to my shopping list?

Raisins, dried apricots, dried apples—all those lusciously sweet dried fruits are delicious, and a good idea added to cereals or tossed in salads. Not only that, they're packed with fruity nutrients. Minerals like iron, copper and potassium. Vitamins too (though vitamin C is often lost.) That's the good news. Everything else is concentrated too, including the calories. Eat in small amounts. If you are allergic to sulfites, avoid dried fruits such as raisins, prunes and peaches, which may have sulfites added to prevent browning. Look for sulfite-free varieties.

Peeled, cut and bagged veggies are so convenient. Am I losing out on nutrients?

When you're stuck for time, this is a wonderful way to save minutes in the kitchen without much loss in nutrients. The downside? Pre-packaged veggies do cost a bit more. Make sure that you buy fresh produce, refrigerate it and eat by the "best before" date.

How can I protect my family from pesticide residues in fruit and vegetables?

- Buy local produce.
- Eat what is in season.
- Choose a variety to minimize your exposure to any one pesticide.
- Unless you're going to peel them, scrub all fruit and vegetables and rinse thoroughly.
- Peel oranges and grapefruit with a knife; do not bite into peel.
- Throw away the outer leaves of leafy vegetables such as lettuce and cabbage and the leaves at the top of vegetables such as celery and cauliflower.
- Peel waxed fruit and vegetables when possible. Although safe in themselves, waxes seal in fungicide or pesticide residues.

Organic foods

In Canada, foods that say "organically grown" or "certified organic" must meet standards set by government and local independent agencies. Buying organic produce is a vote for a certain kind of agriculture that replenishes the soil, and protects the water supply and the people who work in the fields. Many people believe that organic foods offer extra nutrition. To be honest, we don't know. The nutrient content of a food is determined more by its genes, the climate, when it was picked and how it was shipped and stored than by the type of fertilizer used or soil in which it was grown.

Organic foods often cost more, and the produce may not look perfect, but those who do buy organic say that the flavour is better. It's a personal choice—and an environmentally friendly decision.

Fresh fruit and vegetables contain essential nutrients that may actually help your body resist disease, prevent cancer and resist the ravages of chemical pollution. Organic or not, eat plenty of fruit and vegetables.

Spinach? Yuck!

You can't force kids to eat foods they don't like, but you can persuade them—subtly. If they're old enough, suggest that they help you prepare the vegetables for supper. (Even little ones can have fun tearing up lettuce leaves for a family salad.) When you've actually peeled the carrots yourself, it's tough to say no when they show up on your plate. Speaking of carrots, kids usually prefer vegetables that are brightly coloured and crunchy. Carrots, of course, but also red pepper strips, snow peas, broccoli flowers, new green beans, the list goes on. Kids often prefer their vegetables raw—less work for you! Served up on a platter with a creamy low-fat dip, they're much more fun.

Tell your kids they're going skinny-dipping! Just mix equal parts of low-fat mayonnaise and low-fat yogurt, and season to taste with ketchup or powdered soup mix.

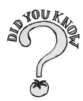

• Cruciferous vegetables are said to help in protecting against certain forms of cancer. Cruciferous comes from the word "cross." These vegetables have a cross-shaped flower. They include cabbage, broccoli, brussels sprouts, cauliflower, kohlrabi (that vegetable that looks like a sputnik), kale and turnips.

Here's a tip to help fruit ripen faster. Don't put fruit out in the sun because heat and light can cause nutrient loss. Instead, punch some holes in a brown paper bag, put the fruit inside and leave it in a cool place. Adding an apple or kiwi fruit to the bag also speeds up the ripening process. They give off ethylene, a natural gas that causes fruit to ripen. In fact, this gas is often used to ripen fruit on its way from orchard to table. It isn't harmful. Because of this ripening action, apples and kiwi fruit need to be kept away from fruit that is already at its peak. Keeping fruit in the fridge will slow the ripening process.

Veg out whenever you can

Fresh vegetables are a wonderfully easy way to boost your fibre and vitamin intake. And you can't beat them for value. Buy vegetables in season when they're at their peak. That way, you'll get maximum flavour. And use them fresh.

The closer a vegetable is grown to your home, the better it usually tastes. After all, you know how you feel after three or four days on the road! Preparing salad greens night after night can be a chore. Instead, why not do the basics as soon as you unpack your shopping? Wash lettuce and other greens. Store them in plastic bags (with a paper towel added to absorb any moisture). Then tear into pieces when you need them. What you might lose in vitamin C you will save in time. Your choice.

If you are trying to manage your weight, veggies are the secret. Relatively low in calories, they're a great way to have a second helping without feeling deprived. Be creative. Snack on crisp celery or carrot sticks with low-fat dips. Build bountiful vegetable salads. Whisk up tasty homemade soups. Steam, roast or bake your veggies. In short, include them whenever you can.

Is it fresh?
How to give veggies the eye!

Artichokes Look for those with tightly closed leaves and no bruises. Squeeze them. Fresh artichokes squeak.

Asparagus Bright green stalks with closed pointed tips are at their peak. Cold water or refrigeration keeps them fresh in the super-market. You do the same.

Avocado Flawless skin is what you want. If hard, leave to ripen on the counter. If soft, store in the fridge. Remember, avocado is high in fat, but it is the healthy monounsaturated fat.

Beans Buy them loose if you can and pick out those with bright colour and velvety feel. If they're full of beans, forget 'em. They'll be old and tough.

Beets Full and firm is what you're looking for. Try to buy them with the greens attached. Steam and serve those separately for a nutritional jumpstart.

Bok Choy   Also called Chinese mustard cabbage. Stalks should be firm and white, topped with deep green, veined leaves. Cooking cuts the sharp tang of the leaves and sweetens the stalks.

Broccoli   Stalks should look tender and crisp and should snap easily. Florets should be green—the darker the better. Yellow means they're "past it". Cook fast to cut down on cooking smells. Keep the beta-carotene-rich leaves for your soup pot.

Brussels sprouts   Deeply coloured, tightly packed leaves mean freshness. Any little holes? A worm got there first.

Cabbage   Green or red, choose firm and heavy heads with tightly closed leaves. As with brussels sprouts, watch for evidence of worms.

Carrots   Leave limp, pale carrots in the bin. Chop off any tops before you put them away so they can't draw moisture away from the carrots.

Cauliflower   White, firm, clean looking florets and bright green leaves mean freshness.

Celery   Choose firm, tightly closed bunches with light green leaves. Dark green celery is often stringy.

Corn   Pull back the husk and check for plump, firm, tightly packed kernels.

Cucumber   Look for bright green colour and firmness. Watch for shrivelled ends.

Eggplant   The skin should be as smooth as dark purple satin. Firm, heavy eggplants are your best choice. Leave behind any with soft spots or bruises. A small "navel" at the bottom means fewer seeds inside.

Garlic   Heads should be firm and heavy with no green sprouts or soft spots.

Greens   For cooking greens like kale, chard and mustard greens, pick the freshest looking leaves you can find and ones as vividly coloured as possible. Remove the outside leaves.

For salad greens, rinse and dry them well and store in your vegetable crisper until needed, in moisture-proof bags with a paper towel added.

Mushrooms Look for tightly closed caps with no soft or bruised areas. Store in a paper bag. Plastic will make them mushy.

Onions The firmer, the better. Soft spots or green sprouts mean an onion is past its prime.

Peppers Pick the firmest peppers you can find in the darkest colours. The walls should feel thick.

Potatoes Not a good buy if the skin is shrivelled, soft or green, or if the potatoes are sprouting. Store in a brown paper bag or dark cupboard at room temperature, not in the fridge where their starch will turn to sugar and alter the taste. Cut away any green areas before cooking but eat the skin whenever possible.

Squash (summer) Thin-skinned and tender, zucchini and baby squash taste sweetest when they're small or medium sized. Look for plump, firm, heavy squash with a bright, uniform colour.

Spinach Look for small leaves, thin stems and a bright green colour. Should smell sweet, not musty.

Squash (winter) Rich in beta carotene (vitamin A), acorn, butternut, spaghetti and pumpkin are just a few of this gloriously colourful family. Look for deep colour and smooth rinds free of cracks. Weigh them in your hand—they should feel heavy. Stored in a cool, dark place, winter squash will last for several weeks.

Sui Choy You may know this as Chinese cabbage or Napa cabbage. Either way, it should be compact and barrel shaped with white, crunchy stalks and crinkly, pale green leaves.

Sweet potatoes Smooth skin with no wrinkles is what you want. Check that the ends aren't discoloured. Root vegetables are sweeter when smaller.

Tomatoes Choose them one by one so you can look for firm, plump tomatoes that aren't overripe or blemished. Keep them out on the counter, not in the refrigerator.

Turnips Small means sweet. Firm and smooth skinned means the best flavour.

• Double your fibre intake by eating potatoes with the skin on.

• Instead of stir-frying vegetables in oil, try sautéing them in a little stock or low-fat salad dressing.

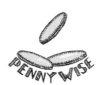

Seven ways to get the most nutrients for your money

1. Prepare fruits and vegetables just before you cook them.
2. Cook vegetables with the skin on.
3. Steam, roast or microwave produce.
4. Cook produce as briefly as possible.
5. Cook large chunks rather than small pieces.
6. Cover and refrigerate juices after opening.
7. Eat raw fruits and vegetables whenever you can.

fun food...fast

Veggie power

Colourful Coleslaw
Mix together thinly sliced red and green cabbage, raisins, chopped apple and a few chopped walnuts. Toss with a mixture of equal parts low-fat mayonnaise and low-fat yogurt.

Sweet Carrots
Steam carrots until tender-crisp. Toss with orange juice and honey and cook until they have a glazed look. Another time, try a mixture of orange marmalade with lemon juice and a dab of margarine. It explodes with flavour.

Nutty Cauliflower
Sauté florets in broth or water and toss with parsley and sliced toasted almonds.

Perfect Corn
Add sugar to the cooking water to enhance the sweetness. Salt toughens the kernels.

Eggplant Secrets Cracked Open
Eggplants absorb oil like a sponge. Reduce the fat you need by broiling or grilling instead of sautéing them. Cut lengthwise into thick slices—there's no need to peel them—prick with a fork and brush with a mixture of oil, chopped garlic and herbs. Turn the slices as they brown.

Need skinless eggplant? Leave whole, or halve the eggplant lengthwise, prick it all over with a fork, place cut side down and broil until skin is blistered and blackened. Place in a paper bag for a few minutes and the skin will peel off easily.

Great English Cucumbers
Just grate them into a bowl, squeeze to remove moisture and add low-fat yogurt, dill, minced garlic and salt to taste.

Homemade Sun-dried Tomatoes
Place sliced tomatoes in a single layer on a cookie sheet. Bake at 400°F (200°C) for about eight minutes or until lightly browned and crisp. Store in a jar in the fridge. A wonderful addition to pasta sauces (and only you have to know they weren't dried in the sun).

Oven-roasted Vegetables
Cut eggplant, peppers, mushrooms, butternut squash or zucchini into one-inch (2.5 cm) cubes and toss with a mixture of olive oil, garlic and herbs—try balsamic vinegar too. Place skin side up on a baking sheet and roast at 400°F (200°C) until browned, 15 to 30 minutes. Shake the pan a few times as the vegetables cook to prevent sticking. The result? Vegetables with intense flavour, crisp skin and tender flesh.

Use as a salad on crisp lettuce, toss them with pasta or spread on a pizza crust with salsa, low-fat cheese and a sprinkle of parmesan.

Ratatouille
A wonderfully tasty dish originating in France. Sauté large chunks of unpeeled eggplant, tomato, onion, red or green peppers, zucchini and some chopped garlic in a little olive oil. Season with basil, thyme and oregano. Cover and let simmer in its juices for 30 minutes. Make lots. Ratatouille is terrific hot or cold. It can be whizzed in the blender for a fast homemade soup—and it freezes beautifully.

Quick Tomato Salad

Mix chopped tomato, chopped onion and cubed low-fat mozzarella. Drizzle with red wine vinegar and vegetable oil. How's that for simple?

Low-fat French "Fries"

Cut large potatoes into wedges and brush lightly with oil. Sprinkle with basil or paprika. Layer on baking sheet sprayed with nonstick cooking spray or lined with parchment paper. Bake at 450°F (230°C) for 40 minutes. Turn as required.

Great Broiled Potatoes

Cut potatoes in quarters, leaving skins on for increased nutritional value. Microwave for a few minutes until almost cooked. Toss in low-fat Italian dressing. Broil for 2–3 minutes. Turn and broil again. Drizzle with more dressing and serve. Yum!

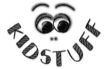

Ant Logs

Kids love these as a snack! Fill celery stalks with peanut butter and sprinkle with raisins.

Quick! Name the vegetable most North American kids eat most.

The answer? Potatoes. Made into french fries.

Too bad, because then they are loaded with fat. One large potato weighs in at only 180 calories. Turn that potato into french fries and its calorie count rockets to over 600. Check above for low-fat "fries" that kids will love.

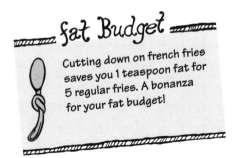

Fat Budget

Cutting down on french fries saves you 1 teaspoon fat for 5 regular fries. A bonanza for your fat budget!

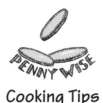

Cooking Tips

The longer you boil vegetables, the more vitamins you lose. Steam or microwave vegetables whenever you can and save the water for adding to soups and stocks.

Storage Tips

- Keep most fruit in the fridge to stop the process of ripening. Kiwi fruits and apples produce ethylene gas which will cause the fruit around them to ripen faster. Keep them both separate from other fruit and vegetables—unless you want this effect.
- Refrigerate green leafy vegetables in vegetable crisper or in moisture-proof bags with a paper towel added.
- Potatoes, carrots, sweet potatoes and other root vegetables keep best in a cool and moist place (not the fridge) to prevent withering.
- Quick, before they go bad, freeze leftover raw vegetables for use in soups and stocks.
- Don't let root vegetables wither away. Buy carrots, parsnips, beets, turnips and other cold-weather favourites without their tops, or cut away the greens when you get home. The green leaves look pretty but they suck nutrients and moisture from the roots—the part you want to eat. Save beet greens to steam, or to chop and add to soups or pastas.

fun food...fast

Five ways to give potatoes a-peel

We know that the usual blobs of butter or sour cream aren't a good idea. No problem. Here are five healthy ways to dress up a potato.

- Top baked potatoes with salsa or fat-free sour cream or low-fat yogurt seasoned with flavoured vinegar, parsley, green onions.
- Sprinkle new potatoes with chopped green onions, chives, fresh dill or rosemary.
- Grind some black pepper and add a few drops of sesame oil for an intriguing Asian twist, or add just a few drops of lower-salt soy sauce.
- Try a dab of low-fat margarine mixed with lemon juice or Dijon mustard.
- Blend soup stock or wine into mashed potatoes, plus puréed cooked vegetables. Try broccoli, asparagus and zucchini for starters.

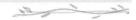

Put the squeeze on fresh fruit

Buying fruits loose rather than bagged lets you choose each one individually.

Apples If you can dent it with your finger, don't buy it.

Bananas They ripen with time, so buy as you need them—green for later in the week, ripe for snacking while you unpack.

Berries If the box is damp or stained, look for another one. It means that the bottom layers of fruit are decaying. Buy uncrushed berries with no mould. Buy strawberries loose if you can and choose each one individually.

Cherries Buy them ripe and avoid any sticky ones. They will damage the others.

Grapefruit Firm and springy is what you're looking for. Weigh one against another in your hands. Thin-skinned ones that feel heavy for their size are juicier.

Grapes If they look plump and good enough to eat, they are. Stems should be green and supple.

Kiwi Press them gently. If they yield, they're ripe.

Lemons and Limes Choose firm, plump ones that are heavy for their size, rich in colour and have a slightly glossy skin.

Mangoes Choose firm and unblemished fruit that smell sweet and yield to gentle pressure. Note: wash your hands after touching mangoes; they contain a chemical that you may be sensitive to.

Melons: Honeydew and Cantaloupe Look for dull, velvety skin. Then check the top. A sunken, smooth scar means they were picked ripe. The bottom should yield slightly to pressure. Smell the aroma. You can buy melons underripe too and let them ripen at room temperature.

Nectarines Pick plump nectarines that are slightly soft along the seam. Hard, green nectarines may not ripen.

Oranges	Choose ones that are firm, heavy and free from spots and wrinkles.
Papayas	Look for those that are mostly yellow and have a pleasant smell. Press them gently. They should give slightly, but shouldn't feel soft.
Peaches	A distinct peachy aroma and slightly soft fruit is what you're looking for. Buy peaches as you want to eat them, ripe or nearly ripe. Once off the tree, they won't ripen any more.
Pears	Pick firm, unbruised pears that yield to pressure. Colour doesn't matter. You can even buy them green and let them ripen at room temperature.
Pineapples	Squeeze them gently with your fingertips. They should give a little.
Plums	Think plump and slightly soft with perfect skins. Buy them ripe.
Rhubarb	Choose firm, crisp stalks and chop off the leaves.
Watermelon	At its best when the surface is smooth with a dullish sheen and the underside is a creamy yellow. Its ends should yield slightly when you press them. The final test? Slap it. A dull, flat sound means an underripe watermelon. A hollow noise tells you it's past its best.

- Fruit gets sweeter with age. Vegetables get starchy. As fruit matures, its starch is converted into sugar. As vegetables mature, the sugar turns into starch, and they become drier and mealier.

Buying juice? Choose products labelled "juice," otherwise you may be buying expensive fruit-flavoured sugar water.

If pineapples are all the same price but different sizes, pick the biggest one. Their skin is all the same thickness so you'll get more fruit for your money.

fun food...fast

Simple sunny fresh fruit

Granny Smith's Best Baked Apples

This homey dessert will fill your kitchen with the wonderful aroma of melted cinnamon and brown sugar. The best apple variety to use is Granny Smith.

Core the apple, fill with a mixture of cinnamon, a small amount of sugar and raisins. Place in a baking dish, add a little water, cover and bake at 350°F (180°C) for 30 minutes. Remove cover and bake for 30 minutes longer.

Note: to help apples keep their shape while cooking, run a knife around the middle of each one so that it just breaks the skin before you core and stuff them.

Grapes 'n' Yogurt

Mix low-fat yogurt, a sprinkle of lemon juice and a dash of brown sugar. Stir in green or purple grapes. Chill and let flavours blend.

Hot Pear Delicacy

Sauté sliced, unpeeled pears in fruit juice. Add a pinch of cinnamon, nutmeg or ginger—your choice. Serve immediately with a scoop of fruit-flavoured sherbet.

Apricots on the BBQ

A terrific summer side dish. Just thread pitted fresh apricots on wooden skewers (which you've soaked for half an hour so they don't burn). Brush them lightly with a little melted brown sugar or honey and barbecue for about three minutes. Turn them over, baste them again and cook until soft.

Fruit-on-a-Stick

Made in seconds, this dessert is an easy way to encourage your family to eat more fruit. Simply skewer melon cubes and whole strawberries on a stick. Try banana chunks, peach slices or halved plums too. Whatever takes your fancy. Use low-fat vanilla yogurt as a dip.

Perfect Papaya Dressing

Easy enough to serve the family but fancy enough to wow your friends. Blend chunks of papaya and a few papaya seeds (yes, you can eat them) with the simple balsamic vinaigrette (see page 120). Toss it over a bowl of torn greens—the darker the better—and your salad is ready.

Frozen Bananas

My kids used to love these snack treats when they were young—and they're a great way to use your bananas if they've ripened before you're ready to eat them. All you do is slice bananas into thick chunks, and freeze individually in plastic wrap. Eat frozen.

Moustache Drink

If mornings are crazy, drink breakfast! As delicious as a milkshake—but healthier.

Place a banana, half a cup of low-fat milk and a dash of vanilla in the blender. Add fresh or frozen fruit if you like. Buzz mixture for 30 seconds. Kids will love the moustache they get from drinking it.

TV Frozen Berries Treat

Picking ripe berries at a local farm is one of our favourite summer outings. We enjoy them right away, but we always freeze a bunch for winter nibbles. Just spread them on a cookie sheet in a single layer and leave in the freezer overnight. Then pop them in a plastic bag. They can last for months—although ours rarely do. Try them straight from the bag, or add them to the Moustache Drink. Too late to pick your own? You'll find summer's crop of raspberries, strawberries and blueberries in your supermarket freezer all year round.

Veggies and fruit at a glance

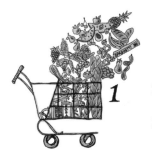

1. Fill your shopping cart with a variety of fruit and vegetables. They're rich in nutrients, a good source of fibre and low in fat (except avocados and olives).
2. Purchase locally grown fruit in season for peak freshness and best value.
3. Frozen fruit and vegetables are good choices when fresh produce is out of season.

Section 2
of your shopping cart

Milk Products

Meat and Alternatives

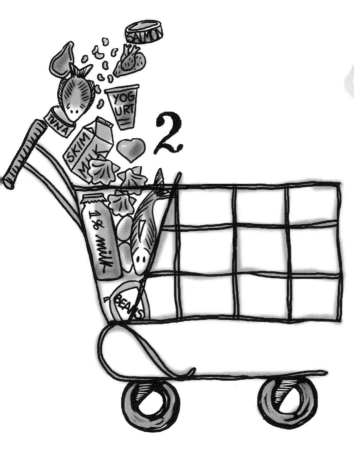

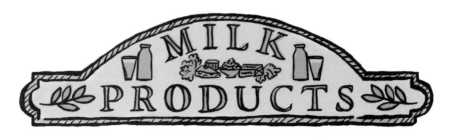

Be deliberate about how you fill the smaller #2 part of your cart, choosing lower-fat milk products.

S hopping cart shoppers, slow down. We're now in the #2 part of your cart, the milk products part, and here's where you have to think a little more carefully about what you choose. Milk is a highly nutritious food packed with vital nutrients essential for good health. Protein, carbohydrates, many vitamins and minerals, milk has a lot! Even when we get too grown-up for milk and cookies, it's still important that we get enough milk. But whole milk and products made from it also contain a lot of saturated fat and cholesterol. That's why they belong in the smaller #2 part of the Heart-Smart™ shopping cart.

Although it's fine to indulge in whole grains, vegetables and fruits to our heart's content, we need to take a slightly longer look at the milk products we pack in our cart. Fortunately, for the HeartSmart shopper, that's easy. Once the fat is skimmed, you have a HeartSmart choice. Take a good look through the dairy case and you'll find manufacturers have responded to our requests for lower-fat foods. These days, whole milk is far from being our only choice. Lower-fat varieties of milk, yogurt and cheese abound. By knowing some simple facts about milk products, we can make a dairy case for the best nutrition!

Milk: the big pitcher

Canada's Food Guide to Healthy Eating recommends at least 2 servings per day. But, depending on our age and stage in life, we may need more.

Children 4–9: 2–3 servings
Youth 10–16: 3–4 servings
Adults: 2–4 servings
Pregnant and breast-feeding women: 3–4 servings

One serving means:
  1 cup (250 mL) milk   1" x 1" x 3" (50 g) cheese
  2 slices (50 g) processed cheese   3/4 cup (175 mL) yogurt

Fat budgeting with milk products

Many milk products may be higher in fat, but lower-fat choices are widely available. That's why you need to think about fat budgeting before filling up the #2 part of your cart. Check the fat budget list and decide how you want to spend your fat budget.

fat Budget

Milk products:

0 tsp fat
skim milk
skim milk yogurt

½ tsp fat
1 cup (250 mL) 1% milk
1 cup (250 mL) buttermilk

1 tsp fat
2 tbsp (25 mL) parmesan cheese
1/4 cup (50 mL) lower-fat ricotta
1 cup (250 mL) 2% milk
1 cup (250 mL) 2% cottage cheese

2 tsp fat
1" x 1" x 3" (50 g) part-skim milk cheese
1/2 cup (125 mL) plain ice cream
1 cup (250 mL) whole milk
1 cup (250 mL) 4.5% cottage cheese
1 cup (250 mL) yogurt with added cream

4 tsp fat
1" x 1" x 3" (50 g) hard cheese

1 teaspoon fat = approximately 5 grams of fat.
These numbers are averages.

HeartSmart Tip

The fat in milk products is mostly saturated—a good reason to budget fat and choose the skimmed options.

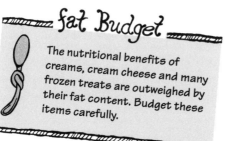

Fat Budget

The nutritional benefits of creams, cream cheese and many frozen treats are outweighed by their fat content. Budget these items carefully.

To find out what nutrients milk products offer and where they fit in the total nutrition picture, see Appendix, page 144.

What about milk and calcium?

Milk products are key sources of dietary calcium. We all need it, and women need it especially. Today one in four of us can expect to develop osteoporosis by the time we're 60. Consuming enough calcium helps build strong bones.

As well as calcium, milk contains vitamin D, which helps calcium absorption. Milk also contains phosphorus, which works with calcium to build bone.

Five steps to stave off osteoporosis

1. Consume enough calcium.
2. Get enough vitamin D.
3. Cut down on caffeine, salt and excessive protein.
4. Manage your weight—being underweight puts you at risk.
5. Do weight-bearing activities such as walking, hiking or dancing.

How much calcium is enough?

Adults need at least 1000 mg daily, and women need up to 1500 mg after menopause. If you are pregnant or nursing you should consume up to 1200 mg daily. Growing teens need a minimum 1200 mg. (To find out how much *you* are getting, see Calcium, page 83.)

What about vitamin D?

Vitamin D helps to absorb calcium. We need more as we get older. If you do not drink milk or fortified soy beverages, consider taking a calcium supplement with vitamin D, especially in the winter.

Look for this health claim on foods that are good or excellent sources of calcium and vitamin D: "A healthy diet with adequate calcium and vitamin D, and regular physical activity help to achieve strong bones and may reduce the risk of osteoporosis."

Calcium? You've got it in the bag

Each of the following contains roughly 300 mg of calcium. How much calcium are *you* consuming daily?

- 1 cup (250 mL) milk*
- 3/4 cup (175 mL) yogurt*
- 1 1/2 oz cheese (45 g)*
- 2 cups (500 mL) cottage cheese*
- 1 cup calcium-fortified soy beverage
- 7 sardines with bones
- 1/2–3/4 can salmon with bones
- 1/2 cup (125 mL) almonds**
- 1 1/2 cups (375 mL) sesame seeds**
- 2–3 cups baked beans***
- 3 cups (750 mL) broccoli***

* Choose skimmed versions whenever possible.

** While you can use almonds and sesame seeds to boost your calcium intake, they're too high in fat to be realistically considered as a source.

***Can't eat this much? Combine with another source of calcium.

Cutting fat without cutting milk

Thanks to the lower-fat milk products that abound, it's easy. Look for the % M.F. (milk fat) or % B.F. (butterfat) on the label and choose products with the lowest percentage of fat. Start by buying 2% instead of whole milk. Move down the fat scale to 1%. Try diluting 1% with skim for a week or two to gradually get yourself and your family used to skim milk.

Less fat doesn't mean less nutrition. You'll still be taking in all that valuable calcium. And by law milk must be fortified with fat-soluble vitamins A and D to replace any that are lost in the skimming process.

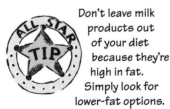

ALL STAR TIP

Don't leave milk products out of your diet because they're high in fat. Simply look for lower-fat options.

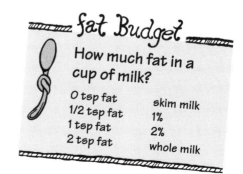

Fat Budget

How much fat in a cup of milk?

0 tsp fat	skim milk
1/2 tsp fat	1%
1 tsp fat	2%
2 tsp fat	whole milk

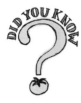

Beware—specialty coffees don't carry labels. But the fat and calories can really add up. In a 12-ounce cup (medium size in most coffee shops), you get on average:

Beverage (12 ounces/375 mL)	Calories	Teaspoons of fat
caffe mocha	450	5
latte with whole milk	200	2.5
latte with skim milk	120	0
black coffee	0	0

fat Budget

A glass at lunch and another at supper? Switching from homogenized milk to skim milk can save you 28 teaspoons of fat a week.

Milk math can be puzzling—2% milk actually contains 35% calories from fat. This is because the number refers to the percentage by weight, not calories, and much of the weight is water. But don't be alarmed. While experts recommend a diet that derives no more than 30% calories from fat, this is a guide for your food intake over an entire day or even a week. It need not be applied to individual foods. Use percentages to compare products. For milk, consider use. In tea or coffee, 2% milk is fine. You're only adding a spoonful or two. If you're pouring milk on your cereal or into a glass, 1% or skim milk is a better choice.

Label Smarts

The percentage of fat that appears on a label usually refers to the percentage of fat by weight, not by calories. Use this percentage to compare products, not to judge the actual fat content.

For the teen who *dislikes* milk

The problem is that your 15-year-old thinks milk is fattening. And, when you're growing up, you're often more concerned with how your body looks than what nutrients you're feeding it. Simply telling your son or daughter that milk is "good" for them probably won't work. Explaining the facts may.

Point out that they're making a great investment in their future health. Encourage them to consume skimmed dairy products, which are low in fat and calories but loaded with nutrition. Mention that one 8-ounce glass (250 mL) of skim milk has only 90 calories—compared with the 150 calories in a 12-ounce can (375 mL) of pop.

DID YOU KNOW?

Even if you're lactose intolerant, there are still ways you can get the goodness of milk.

Add drops or tablets of lactase enzyme to your milk, or buy pretreated milk, or take pills containing the lactase enzyme.

Pick firm cheeses such as cheddar, edam and gouda which are virtually lactose free. But watch your fat budget!

Choose yogurt or buttermilk, which contains live bacterial cultures that help you digest lactose more easily.

Try drinking milk "little and often" with meals throughout the day.

Tips to boost milk intake

- Add low-fat milk to soups instead of water.
- Make tasty drinks using low-fat milk as a base.
- Add powdered milk to soups and drinks.
- Make hot cereals with low-fat milk instead of water.
- Drink a lower-fat latte for your mid-afternoon snack.

Q&A

Which is better, bottles, cartons or pouches?

Nutritionally, there's no difference. Choose whichever you like.

Powdered, evaporated, sterilized, condensed…what's the difference?

Usually found in boxes near the flour and sugar in supermarkets, *skim milk powder* is a great low-fat choice. Keep some in your desk to add to your coffee if your office doesn't have a refrigerator. Add it to milkshakes, mashed potatoes, casseroles and cereals to bump up the nutrition. It has 70 mg of calcium per tablespoon and only 15 calories.

Available whole or skimmed, *canned evaporated milk* is handy to keep in your cupboard. It is found in the baking aisle as it's mostly used for baking. Evaporated milk is made by removing more than half the water in milk. It is fortified with vitamins A and D.

UHT milk is 2% milk treated at high temperatures. It can be stored at room temperature until opened and it still tastes like "real" milk.

Sweetened condensed milk at a whopping 1000 calories per cup breaks all the rules. As with evaporated milk, water is removed, but a large amount of sugar is added too.

A glass of milk will send you off to dreamland faster than counting sheep. It's not just an old wives' tale. Milk contains tryptophan, an amino acid that research has linked to helping us sleep. Try lower-fat milk with a teaspoon of honey and a dash of cinnamon.

What about goat's milk?

Tangy goat's milk contains most of the same nutrients as regular milk, including lactose, but it is higher in fat, and you rarely find lower-fat versions. Some people think it is easier to digest than cow's milk, but there are no studies to prove this.

Do creams and non-dairy coffee lighteners belong in a HeartSmart cart?

Their fat content outweighs any nutritional benefits. Budget carefully.

What about chocolate milk in the kids' lunchboxes?

Nutritionally, it's the same as ordinary milk. The milk is usually lower in fat—2% or 1% milk fat (M.F.). But the chocolate syrup added, though low in fat, boosts the calories. You can make your own by adding chocolate milk mix or syrup to milk. If growing kids won't drink plain milk, give 'em chocolate milk.

Mystical magical yogurt

We've all heard the tales of Hunzas who live to be 120 years old and credit their age to a daily dose of yogurt. Cleopatra was said to have bathed in yogurt because it did wonderful things for her skin.

Promises, promises...Research shows that yogurt is useful in preventing and treating various intestinal problems such as diarrhea, but the nutritional truth is that yogurt is merely milk curdled by the addition of bacteria. It is certainly nutritious, but only as nutritious as its source, milk. It's a good source of calcium, protein and riboflavin but it may also hide fat and calories. Fortunately, your supermarket cooler is loaded with choices.

Check the fat. It's easy.

The yogurt container will tell you how much B.F. (butterfat) or M.F. (milk fat) it contains. The amount depends on which type of milk it is made from. It can range from a low 0.1 % (yogurt made from skim milk, 0 teaspoons fat) to as high as 10% (with added cream, 2 teaspoons fat) per serving. Select the lowest fat you can find.

Watch out for yogurt-covered nuts and raisins. Despite their name, these candies are not a good source of yogurt. The coating is merely a mixture of oil, sugar and yogurt powder.

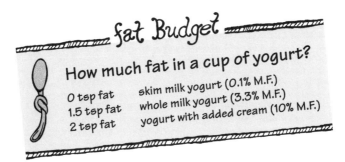

How much fat in a cup of yogurt?

0 tsp fat	skim milk yogurt (0.1% M.F.)
1.5 tsp fat	whole milk yogurt (3.3% M.F.)
2 tsp fat	yogurt with added cream (10% M.F.)

What about those drinkable yogurts that kids love?

A healthy choice for the lunchbox.
Unfortunately, they can be pricey.

Label Smarts

Low-fat yogurt alert! It may not be as low in calories as you think. Adding fruit, fruit sauces or sundae ingredients adds calories. Read labels to compare products.

Why do some lower-fat yogurts taste creamier?

Maybe that's skim milk powder you're tasting. Some manufacturers add it to make yogurt thicker and richer-tasting. It also boosts calcium and protein content without adding fat. You can do the same trick at home. Make your skim milk taste richer by adding 1 to 2 tablespoons skim milk powder to each cup.

Boost your yogurt intake

- Add yogurt to cold soup.
- Use yogurt as a base for veggie dips.
- Make yogurt salad dressings.

fun food...fast

Yummy yogurt ideas

Turn Yogurt into Cheese

Want the creaminess and richness of sour cream or cream cheese without the fat? Place low-fat yogurt in a cheesecloth-lined strainer over a bowl, or in a paper coffee filter in its holder. (Check that the yogurt doesn't contain gelatin or it won't strain.) Let it drain in the fridge to the consistency you want: a couple of hours for creamy, overnight for solid. Discard the whey that drips into the bowl. What remains is low-fat, versatile yogurt cheese, which can be used in so many ways.

Baked Potatoes

Top with yogurt cheese and chopped chives.

Vinaigrette

Substitute 2 parts yogurt cheese for 1 part oil.

Middle Eastern Bruschetta

Spread thin layer of yogurt cheese on toasted bread. Top with thinly sliced tomato, drizzle of olive oil and chopped mint.

Dessert

Sweeten yogurt or yogurt cheese with frozen fruit juice concentrates.

Fruit Dip

Mix 1 cup (250 mL) yogurt cheese with 1 teaspoon (5 mL) honey and a dash of cinnamon, grated nutmeg and grated orange rind.

Skinny Dipping with Yogurt

Low-fat yogurt or yogurt cheese makes a great dip. Simply use it in place of mayonnaise or sour cream in your favourite uncooked recipes. Low-fat yogurt plus:

Mexican salsa

Chopped fresh basil and onion

Curry powder and chutney

Honey mustard and dill (a pinch of sugar smooths out the flavour)

Surprise, it's buttermilk!

It sounds high in fat but it isn't. Buttermilk is usually made from lower-fat milk. Read the label.

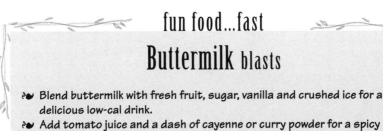

fun food...fast
Buttermilk blasts

- Blend buttermilk with fresh fruit, sugar, vanilla and crushed ice for a delicious low-cal drink.
- Add tomato juice and a dash of cayenne or curry powder for a spicy drink.
- Drizzle over baked potatoes and top with fresh chives.
- Use as a base for cold summer soups.
- Swirl into hot soups at the last minute to enrich them.
- Use in sauces, salad dressings and mashed potatoes.

Be choosy with cheese

It takes 8 pounds of milk to make a pound of cheese. This super-concentrated food is a great source of calcium, but it's high in fat and calories too. A single ounce (30 grams) of hard cheese (the size of a domino) has about 300 mg calcium and 2 teaspoons fat.

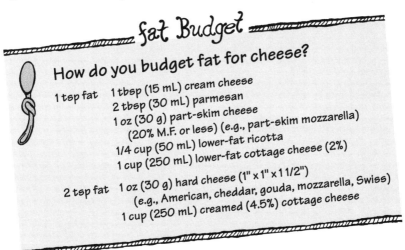

Fat Budget

How do you budget fat for cheese?

1 tsp fat
- 1 tbsp (15 mL) cream cheese
- 2 tbsp (30 mL) parmesan
- 1 oz (30 g) part-skim cheese (20% M.F. or less) (e.g., part-skim mozzarella)
- 1/4 cup (50 mL) lower-fat ricotta
- 1 cup (250 mL) lower-fat cottage cheese (2%)

2 tsp fat
- 1 oz (30 g) hard cheese (1" x 1" x 1 1/2") (e.g., American, cheddar, gouda, mozzarella, Swiss)
- 1 cup (250 mL) creamed (4.5%) cottage cheese

You can lower the fat in your cheese choices by picking lower-fat cottage cheese or part-skim milk ricotta.

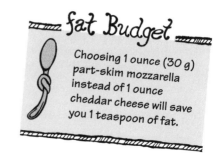

Fat Budget

Choosing 1 ounce (30 g) part-skim mozzarella instead of 1 ounce cheddar cheese will save you 1 teaspoon of fat.

What about goat cheese?

Oops. While goat and sheep's milk cheeses are the rage with gourmets, they're not so popular with the HeartSmart crowd. The reason? High fat. Agreed, feta, Roquefort and chevre are delicious, but use them with caution. A better option? See if low-fat versions are available or use in small amounts.

Buying soy cheese?

Check the Nutrition Facts table for calories, fat and sodium content, and compare. Soy cheese is cholesterol free, but some is made with hydrogenated soy oil. If you have a dairy allergy, beware. Some soy cheeses may have dairy protein such as whey or casein added.

DID YOU KNOW

Vegetarians who substitute cheese for meat may be taking in more fat than they would like. Ounce for ounce, cheese has more calories, saturated fat, cholesterol and sodium than even the fattiest spareribs.

• Low-cholesterol and low-fat cheeses are usually higher in sodium. Salt is added to compensate for the flavour that's lost when the fat is removed. Fat is essential to the taste and texture of cheese. Low-fat cheeses are less creamy and often less tangy.

HeartSmart Tip

Use cheese as an extra for flavouring rather than eating chunks as a snack.

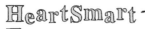

Kids love processed cheese

And it's so handy. Nutritionally, it is marginally lower in protein, vitamin A, calcium and iron, and higher in sodium. Processed cheese is made by melting natural cheese with an emulsifier to form a smooth mass. Pasteurization helps these cheese foods keep longer. Check the label for added ingredients such as cream, and factor those into your buying decision.

Not all dairy products are high in calcium. You need 2 cups cottage cheese or 26 tablespoons of cream cheese to equal the calcium in 1 cup milk.

Always store cheese in foil. Plastic traps moisture which makes cheese mouldy. You can cut mould away from hard cheese but throw soft cheeses out. Mould may have penetrated deep beneath the surface.

We all scream for ice cream

Dutch chocolate, banana fudge, toffee maple...we all have our favourite frozen indulgence. And that's the best way to look at ice cream: as an occasional treat, not as part of your daily diet.

Real ice cream contains 10% milk by weight so ice cream is a good source of calcium with 100–150 mg per 1/2 cup (125 mL) serving. But usually it's high in saturated fat and calories too. If only it didn't taste so good...

Good news...of a kind. One cup ice cream provides almost the same calcium as 1 cup milk! Too bad about the calories. Here's the difference: one cup skim milk contains 90 calories, 1 cup premium ice cream, 350 (ouch!) calories.

The scoop on ice cream

Standard ice cream contains 1–2 teaspoons fat per 1/2 cup (125 mL). Gourmet ice creams may contain twice that amount!

Sherbet usually contains some dairy products as well as fruit.

Frozen dairy desserts such as ice milk are usually made with milk that is skimmed and are therefore lower in fat.

Frozen tofu desserts are dairy free, but they can be high in fat, even though the fat is mostly unsaturated.

Frozen yogurt is made like regular yogurt except that the culturing process is stopped before the characteristic tartness develops. Some varieties are low in fat, but others are made from cream or whole milk. Check the label.

Like it or not, broken cookies, sprinkles, nuts, chocolate chips and crumbled candy bars add extra fat, sugar and calories to your cone or sundae.

What's the real scoop about your favourite frozen desserts? If you are watching your weight, check calories. Brands vary. Sure, many desserts cut fat, but...they may contain added sugar, and be higher in calories than you realize.

Dessert (1/2 cup/125 mL) *	Calories	Teaspoons of fat
ice cream, premium	175	2–3
ice cream, standard	135	1–2
sherbet	135	1/4
low-fat frozen yogurt	125	1/2
sorbet	100	0
ice milk	95	1/4

* Average amounts—check labels

• Watching your weight? Fruit-based sorbets, fruit juice bars or fruit ices are good alternatives to dairy desserts. They are low in calories and contain no fat and no cholesterol. (No calcium either—too bad!) Pick up a pack of moulds from the supermarket and make your own frozen treats for the family
• Choosing frozen tofu? Watch out. It usually has more calories than gourmet ice cream. Look for light versions that are lower in fat and calories.

How much is enough?

When you're reading labels on frozen desserts, remember that a standard serving is 1/2 cup (125 mL)—which is probably less than you think. Measuring it out even once will give you a guideline to go by.

Tricks to make it seem like more? Use smaller bowls or top each serving with fresh fruit or toss with frozen berries. Your dessert will take longer to eat, and have less calories and more healthful nutrients than if you add another scoop.

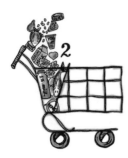

Milk products at a glance

1. Look for milk products low in butterfat (B.F.) or milk fat (M.F.).
2. Choose milk, buttermilk, yogurt and cottage cheese with 2% or less B.F. or M.F.
3. Choose cheeses with 20% or less B.F. or M.F.

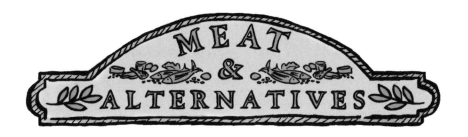

MEAT & ALTERNATIVES

Be deliberate about how you fill the #2 part of your cart, choosing leaner meat, poultry, fish and legumes.

Time to slow down because here's where it gets a bit more complicated. Canada's Food Guide for Healthy Eating groups this eclectic range of foods together because they have one important nutrient in common: protein. But that's where the similarity ends.

Meat products—meat, poultry, fish, eggs—contain cholesterol but don't contain fibre. Plant products such as legumes and peanut butter have no cholesterol but do contain fibre. On top of that, each product has a different amount—and type—of fat. So how do you fill up this #2 part of your cart with nutrition smarts?

To cut the fat, especially the saturated fat, eat leaner meat and trim visible fat. Use lower-fat cooking techniques and marinades to tenderize and add flavour (page 136). Enjoy versatile poultry, choosing white meat cuts with the skin removed. Go big on fish, which is low in saturated fat and high in healthy omega-3s. Add lots of legumes—you won't be stuck for choice!

As more people opt to eat less meat, new products have come on the market. They taste and even look like meat, and have the benefits of fibre, unsaturated fat and other plant-based nutrients. As these foods become more popular, you'll find them in your local supermarket. Look for veggie burgers, hot dogs and chili.

How much do we need?

Canada's Food Guide to Healthy Eating recommends 2–3 servings per day of meat, poultry, fish, eggs or alternatives.

One serving means:
- 1/3 cup (100 g) tofu
- 2 tbsp (30 mL) peanut butter
- 50–100 g meat, poultry or fish
- 1/3–2/3 can (50 g–100 g) canned fish
- 1/2–2/3 cup (125–150 mL) canned beans
- 1–2 eggs

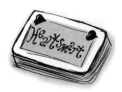

1 serving meat for the average woman =
size of a deck of cards (the size of the
palm of the average woman's hand)

Fat budgeting with meat and alternatives

Meat, poultry, fish, beans, eggs, nuts, seeds—so many options.

Check the fat budget lists below and decide how you want to spend your fat budget.

Fat Budget

Meat and alternatives:

0 tsp fat
dried beans (excluding soybeans), peas, lentils
most white fish
egg white

1/2 tsp fat
90 g canned tuna in water*
3 1/2 oz (100 g) skinless white chicken
  or turkey

1 tsp fat
1 tbsp (15 mL) nuts or seeds*
1 medium egg
1 slice (25 g) salami
3 1/2 oz (100 g) tofu* (amount of fat differs,
  depending on firmness; check label)
3 1/2 oz (100 g) skinless dark chicken
  or turkey
3 1/2 oz (100 g) lean beef, pork, lamb
1 cup (250 mL) chickpeas*
1 cup (250 mL) soy drink*

2 tsp fat
1 small hot dog
3 1/2 oz (100 g) salmon*
3 1/2 oz (100 g) white chicken or turkey
  with skin
3 1/2 oz (100 g) beef, pork, lamb
3 1/2 oz (100 g) extra lean ground beef

	2 tbsp peanut butter*
3 tsp fat	3 1/2 oz (100 g) dark chicken or turkey with skin
	3 1/2 oz (100 g) lean ground beef
	1 cup (250 mL) cooked soybeans*
4 tsp fat	3 1/2 oz (100 g) salami
	3 1/2 oz (100 g) regular ground beef
	3 1/2 oz (100 g) ribs

1 teaspoon fat = approximately 5 grams of fat.
These numbers are averages.
Note that these values are for cooked meats (3 1/2 oz cooked is 4 1/2 oz raw).
* Budget wisely—choose these healthier fats more often.

Look for leaner meats, and select fish and meat alternatives more often.

"HEART AND STROKE FOUNDATION

Health ✓ Check

Label Smarts

You won't find labels on raw meat and poultry (except the ground kind) or on raw fish or seafood.

To find out what nutrients are in meat and alternatives and where they fit in the total nutrition picture, see Appendix, page 144.

Meat: cut it down—no need to cut it out

It's not meat itself that's the problem, it's eating fatty cuts and eating too much of them. It's all about balance.

No question, the trend today is to eat less meat. How times have changed. It used to be that a meal wasn't a meal unless it was meat and potatoes— a big hunk of meat was regarded as a status symbol.

Nutritionists are concerned about total fat and saturated fat, which can be linked to an increased risk of heart disease. But while we need less meat— and protein—than we've grown used to eating, make no mistake: meat does supply important nutrients.

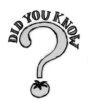

- Eating foods high in dietary cholesterol will not necessarily raise your blood cholesterol, but if your blood cholesterol is high, cut down on your intake of dietary cholesterol (see Appendix page 147).

   - Treat meat as a side dish that complements a meal of veggies, grains or legumes.

   - Avoid eating organ meats (e.g., liver and kidney) where cholesterol and contaminants may be concentrated.

Large amounts of meat don't make you stronger. You can only achieve that by exercising your muscles against resistance. Lift weights, not steaks.

Lean meat shortcuts

The fat content in meat isn't listed on the label. These few simple tips will help you make lower-fat choices in the meat department.

Use your eyes
Look for the leanest meat you can. Cut off all visible fat. The fat you can see marbling some meat cuts—those white streaks—is impossible to remove. Choose those cuts rarely.

Check its speedometer
I'm serious. If an animal can move faster than you, it's lean. Buffalo (bison), deer (venison), rabbit, partridge, pheasant and quail—choose any one of these and you'll win out nutritionally. A lower percentage of fat. Lower in cholesterol. Plus more intense flavour so you'll be satisfied with less. Talk about a win-win situation.

Test your meat cut IQ
Meat from close to the ribs has the most fat. It's logical. The animal needs a fatty layer to protect its vital organs from injury. Cuts to limit are short-ribs, whole ribs and blade roast. Cuts of meat close to the hip usually have the least fat. These areas are on the move. Good choices are cuts such as sirloin tip roast and steaks, eye of the round and tenderloin.

Deal yourself a HeartSmart serving
Keep portions the size of the palm of your hand.

HeartSmart Tip

Meat cuts with the words "round" or "loin" on the label are lean. Good choices.

DID YOU KNOW

Lean ground beef is not necessarily as low in fat as lean cuts of meat.

ALL STAR TIP

Decrease the fat content of ground beef before adding it to chili or spaghetti by browning in a nonstick pan and draining the fat.

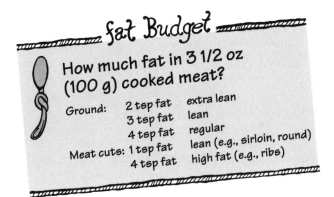

Fat Budget

How much fat in 3 1/2 oz (100 g) cooked meat?

Ground:	2 tsp fat	extra lean
	3 tsp fat	lean
	4 tsp fat	regular
Meat cuts:	1 tsp fat	lean (e.g., sirloin, round)
	4 tsp fat	high fat (e.g., ribs)

What if the meat looks purple?

Meat is red from the myoglobin it contains (an oxygen-storing muscle pigment), not from blood, most of which is removed when the animal is slaughtered. The harder the muscle has worked, the darker the meat colour. That's why chicken and turkey legs are dark while wings and breasts are white.

Meat that is not exposed to oxygen (such as the inside of a roast, or vacuum-packed meat) is dark purple. It needn't affect your choice.

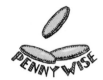

Best meat for your money

- The date on fresh meat refers to the day it was packaged. Fresh meats may be reduced in price 1 to 2 days after that date. Use the same day.
- "Best before" dates are used on processed meats.
- Look for cream-coloured fat that springs when you touch it. Avoid hard yellow fat. Remove all fat once you get it home.
- Exposure to oxygen turns meat brown. It's still edible but you should use it immediately.

 In general, today's meat is leaner. Ranchers are crossbreeding lean with traditional breeds and sending cattle to market younger—and leaner.
More fat is trimmed away at the packing stage before the meat reaches the market.

Pork picks

Pork is leaner than it used to be, and low-fat cuts can be compared to the leanest cuts of beef. Pork fat is lower in saturated fat than beef fat—but it's still not as lean as skinless turkey or chicken breast.

Choose lean cuts with the word "loin" (such as tenderloin, center loin, top loin), lean ham or fresh pork leg.

Limit fattier cuts like spareribs, bacon, regular ground pork and shoulder roast.

Keep portions to the size of the palm of your hand.

 If you are watching your salt intake, limit bacon, ham and cold cuts.

Choosing lamb?

Lean cuts are more tender than similar cuts of beef. Leanest cut? Leg of lamb.

Meat is made of iron

Meat is full of iron—the kind that is more readily absorbed by the body than that found in legumes. Women especially need to be on the watch for iron deficiency. We need to make special efforts to obtain enough iron from our diet. Meat is also a good source of zinc and vitamin B12. If you cut out animal foods, eat lots of legumes, whole grains leavened with yeast, and processed soy products to supply zinc—and take a vitamin B12 supplement.

You'll find iron in these plant foods:

- Legumes: beans, dried peas, and lentils
- Grains and cereal: enriched or fortified products
  e.g., breakfast cereal (cream of wheat, oatmeal), breads, spaghetti
- Fruits: dried apricots, raisins, prunes
- Vegetables: broccoli, bok choy, beet greens
- Others: almonds, sesame seeds, blackstrap molasses

Ironclad tips on plant sources

Iron is better absorbed from animal than vegetable sources, and some vegetables contain substances that hinder absorption. Tables listing the iron content of plant foods only tell half the story.

To increase absorption:
- Consume a vitamin C–containing food (such as a glass of orange juice) with your iron source.
- Eat a small amount of meat or fish at the same time.
- Avoid drinking black or green tea with iron-containing plant sources.
- Cook in cast iron pots.

Cluck-cluck!

Poultry used to be a special Sunday dinner treat. Not any more. Changes in breeding and marketing techniques mean that it's more abundant and affordable than ever. In fact, Canada produces more chicken in 24 hours than was produced in the whole of one year in the 1930s.

Add it to your HeartSmart™ shopping cart and enjoy its versatility—who ever gets tired of eating chicken? Choose turkey too, which is even lower in fat. Not all parts of poultry are low in total fat. Eating the skin more than doubles the amount of fat and saturated fat.

HeartSmart Tip

Chicken has roughly the same amount of cholesterol as red meat but is lower in fat, and the fat is less saturated.

Guide to buying poultry

- Choose white rather than dark meat to get less fat and a little less cholesterol.
- Look for moist, plump poultry—that means it's fresh—and give it a sniff. It should smell clean.
- Frozen poultry should be rock hard. Ice crystals or frozen liquid mean that it has been defrosted and then re-frozen. The result? Loss of flavour.
- Buy ground poultry from a reputable butcher. Sometimes skin is mixed in, which makes it higher in fat than ground beef.

fat Budget

How much fat in half a breast or a whole leg of chicken (3 1/2 oz or 100 g)?

1/2 tsp fat	light meat, no skin
2 tsp fat	light meat with skin
1 tsp fat	dark meat, no skin
3 tsp fat	dark meat with skin

* Measurements are approximate. Turkey has slightly less fat than chicken.

Turning to turkey

Lower in fat than chicken, turkey is an excellent HeartSmart choice. Almost all turkey fat is found in the skin. Just cut it away.

Substitute ground turkey in your favourite ground beef recipes such as burgers or meatballs. Just add bread crumbs, egg white, Worcestershire sauce and mustard.

HeartSmart

Tip Choose 3 1/2 ounces (100 g) light meat without any skin instead of 3 1/2 ounces dark meat with skin and you'll save 2 1/2 teaspoons of fat.

Chicken wings are mostly skin (and a chicken's fat is under its skin). Limit how many you eat.

DID YOU KNOW

How to size up a chicken

You can tell the approximate age of a chicken by pressing against the breastbone. If it's pliable, it's young and tender.

Most chickens sold in the supermarket are broilers (sometimes called fryers). Weighing between 2.5 and 5 pounds (1.2–2.2 kg), they can be roasted, grilled, steamed, sautéed, poached or broiled.

Roasting chickens are big guys, older and larger chickens that weigh up to 6 pounds (2.7 kg). Perfect for a family-sized roast chicken dinner.

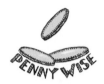

Boneless chicken breast is no more expensive, ounce for ounce, than bone-in. But if you're handy with a knife, buy bone-in and use the bones for stock.

Think twice at the deli counter

Fast for sandwiches, quick in salads, deli meats are the ultimate in convenience. But they're not perfect. In fact they may pack a double whammy of substances that you might not want to feed your family: fat and sodium.

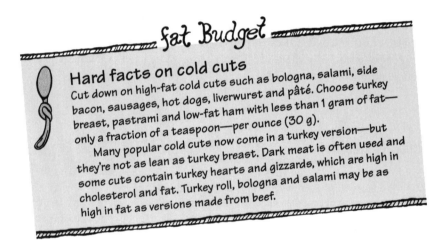

fat Budget

Hard facts on cold cuts

Cut down on high-fat cold cuts such as bologna, salami, side bacon, sausages, hot dogs, liverwurst and pâté. Choose turkey breast, pastrami and low-fat ham with less than 1 gram of fat—only a fraction of a teaspoon—per ounce (30 g).

Many popular cold cuts now come in a turkey version—but they're not as lean as turkey breast. Dark meat is often used and some cuts contain turkey hearts and gizzards, which are high in cholesterol and fat. Turkey roll, bologna and salami may be as high in fat as versions made from beef.

HeartSmart Tip

Limit favourite deli accompaniments such as pickles, olives and sauerkraut. They're high in salt.

The sizzle on sausages

Most sausages are pork based, but they can be made from any kind of chopped ground meat. It's the seasoning that gives Italian sausage or Mexican chorizo its distinctive flavour. Most sausages are high in fat and sodium. They may contain 2–3 teaspoons of fat, depending on size. But you may find lower-fat sausages occasionally. Read the labels and watch that fat budget.

The hot news on hot dogs

Beef, pork, chicken, turkey or tofu—whichever kind you pick, do your homework first. Read the label to check the fat content and keep the following information in mind:

Chicken or turkey dogs may not necessarily be low in fat. If they're made from dark meat and skin, their fat content will be high.

Tofu hot dogs may be leaner and they do offer a nutritional advantage—the fat they contain is unsaturated and they have no cholesterol.

Beware of claims that hot dogs are 90% fat free. This is a measure of fat by weight, not by calories. Check the label to find out the fat content.

Hot diggity dog! Lower-fat hot dogs contain less than 1 teaspoon fat. Regular dogs have two or three times as much. Compare brands and dig into dogs with the least fat, calories and sodium.

Reel in some fish

Seafood is good for you. All kinds. Both fish and shellfish are low in fat and saturated fat. Any fats contained in fish are the healthy omega-3 fatty acids (see Appendix, page 146) that may protect you against heart disease. Most varieties (except for shrimp, squid and caviar) are low in cholesterol too. Load up the #2 part of your shopping cart.

Hook the best

Buy fish last on your trip and store it in its original wrapper in the coldest part of your refrigerator.

Choose steaks and fillets that are moist. Whole fish should have red or bright pink gills and shiny, tightly clinging scales.

Throw fish back if...

- ❧ it smells fishy
- ❧ it's brown or dry around the edges
- ❧ it's covered with ice crystals or has freezer burn

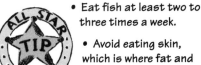

- Eat fish at least two to three times a week.

- Avoid eating skin, which is where fat and contaminants may be concentrated.

fun food...fast

Fish made fabulous

Plain, simple fish is the perfect low-fat choice for a healthy meal. Bake, broil or grill, adding flavour with herbs and lemon or orange juice. Spicy salsas add zest.

To cook whole fish, measure at its thickest part and cook for 10 minutes for every inch. Fish is cooked when it's opaque. Salmon, which is higher in fat than other fish, can be cooked longer without drying out.

To microwave, place fish in microwaveable dish. Season with pepper, lemon juice or herbs (do not add salt until after cooking). Cover with plastic wrap, leaving one corner open to get rid of steam. Cook until fish flakes when tested with a fork.

Fat Budget

Fatty fish, lean fish, they're all HeartSmart. How much fat in 3 1/2 oz (100 g) fresh fish?

0 tsp fat	cod, flounder, haddock, monkfish, pike, pollock, perch, whiting, red snapper, halibut, sole
1 tsp fat	swordfish, fresh bluefin tuna, trout
2 tsp fat	salmon, albacore, mackerel, herring, bluefish

Land fish on your plate for heart health

The fat in fatty fish contains a heart-healthy unsaturated fat called omega-3. It makes platelets in the blood less likely to stick together, which decreases the chance of blood clotting and may help reduce the possibility of a heart attack. Experts say that eating at least two servings a week of fatty fish can protect your heart and blood flow.

Fish-oil supplements are not a substitute for fish. They have potential side effects, may contain contaminants or even lack omega-3 fats, and are definitely missing the nutrients found in whole fish. Remember too that, like any oil, a teaspoon of fish-oil supplement contains roughly 40 calories.

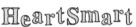

DID YOU KNOW

- The rumours are false! With the exception of shrimp, shellfish are *not* significantly high in cholesterol. While they *do* contain some, the amount is often no higher than chicken or beef (see Appendix, page 147). They are low in fat and a good option—provided you don't serve melted butter on the side.
- Maybe it's just a tall fish tale, but the countries that eat the most fish, such as Japan and Finland, seem to have the lowest rates of depression.

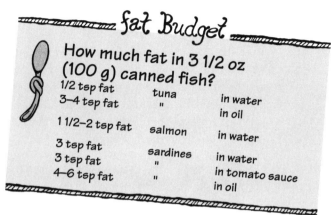

Fat Budget

How much fat in 3 1/2 oz (100 g) canned fish?

1/2 tsp fat	tuna	in water
3–4 tsp fat	"	in oil
1 1/2–2 tsp fat	salmon	in water
3 tsp fat	sardines	in water
3 tsp fat	"	in tomato sauce
4–6 tsp fat	"	in oil

HeartSmart Tip

3 1/2 ounces (100 g) of oil-packed tuna contains 3 to 4 teaspoons of fat before you drain it. Why not choose water-packed tuna instead?

ALL STAR TIP

Boost your calcium intake by eating the bones of canned sardines and salmon.

What about imitation shellfish?

They look like their wealthier crab and lobster cousins but how do these look-alikes cut it nutritionally? The answer is, very well. They're a tasty addition to salads and sandwiches and, at only 100 calories for 3 1/2 ounces (100 g), a wise choice if you're watching your weight.

These pretenders are made mainly from pollock, a deep-sea whitefish that is low in fat and rich in high-quality protein. The filleted fish is ground, then refined to remove its natural colour, flavour and odour. New colour and flavour are added. The results are crab legs, shrimp, scallops and lobster tails that resemble the real thing.

The differences? Imitation shellfish has more sodium and less omega-3 fatty acid. Processing destroys some of the vitamins and minerals.

Where do fish sticks fit?

Be wary. With their batter coating they contain more fat and salt than fresh fish. If you serve them with ketchup and cocktail sauce you also raise your sodium intake. Tartar sauce adds extra fat too. Make your own low-fat version. See recipe on page 135.

Cracking the case for eggs

Egg consumption dropped by over 20% between 1980 and 1990 as North Americans became cholesterol-conscious. Turns out you may not need to cut down on the eggs you eat.

Eggs are a powerhouse of nutrition, and rich in protein, B vitamins, vitamin A and iron. They're economical too, and you can't beat them for versatility.

People are often concerned that eggs are a major source of cholesterol. It's true. A single egg contains about 190 mg dietary cholesterol as well as 1 teaspoon of fat. But remember, it's not so much the cholesterol as the saturated fat in your diet that affects your blood cholesterol. An egg contains less than half a teaspoon of saturated fat (compared with 1 teaspoon in a 3 1/2 ounce [100 g] hamburger patty).

Egg whites don't contain fat or cholesterol. Eat as much as you like. You can successfully switch two egg whites for one whole egg in most recipes—or substitute one whole egg and two egg whites for two whole eggs.

Buying and storing eggs safely

Never purchase eggs that have been sitting at room temperature. Always buy refrigerated eggs, and pop them in the fridge when you get home—not in the egg rack where they are exposed to warm air each time you open the fridge, but on the shelf in their original carton.

Avoid eggs with visible cracks. Before you lift a carton into your cart, jiggle each egg to make sure that it's not stuck to the bottom. It takes time but it's worth it.

Should I limit the eggs I eat?

Maybe. Maybe not.

Most people can eat eggs in moderation without any harmful effects on their blood cholesterol. But limit your intake to two eggs a week if you or your family have high blood cholesterol. You don't have to limit the number of egg whites you use.

Brown eggs or white eggs?

Yolk and shell colour have no bearing on an egg's nutritional quality.

What about egg substitutes?

Made from egg whites, with vegetable oil, flavour and colouring added, these are not necessarily low in fat. The equivalent of one egg may contain as much as 4 grams, almost 1 teaspoon. But the fat is unsaturated and they are cholesterol free.

How can I avoid leftover egg yolks?

Check your supermarket cooler for egg whites available in liquid form. These make a good substitute for fresh eggs and save you the task of separating the yolk from the white—and they spare you the problem of what to do with all those yolks.

What are omega-3 eggs?

Hens fed a diet containing fish oil, algae or flaxseed—all foods rich in omega-3 fats—lay eggs containing this nutrient. These "designer" eggs may also contain more vitamin E, and less cholesterol and fat, than regular eggs.

Meet the legendary legume family

As we continue to fill the #2 part of our shopping cart, it's time to look at legumes (dried beans, peas and lentils). Although they fit happily within the meat group because they are high in protein, their family background is vegetarian.

Legumes are simply the seeds that grow inside the pods of leguminous plants. We know them mostly as dried beans, peas and lentils. A poor man's meat? No way! Inexpensive, yes, but legumes are crammed with nutrition. Consider what they offer. Soluble fibre for starters—the kind that may reduce blood cholesterol. Loads of B vitamins, lots of protein and little fat. To cap it off, they're also a source of calcium, iron and potassium.

They're also versatile and very, very cheap. In truth, they would fit well in the #1 part of your shopping cart.

One cup (250 mL) of most legumes = 200 to 300 calories and 6 to 12 grams fibre.

Are legumes a good source of protein?

Legumes are almost perfect—but not quite. They lack one or more amino acids (protein building blocks). All you do is add the missing amino acid, which you'll find in grains, nuts, seeds or in small amounts of animal foods. Don't even worry about having to eat both at the same meal. As long as they are eaten over the course of the day you'll be doing fine nutritionally.

Buying and cooking
peas, beans and lentils

Supermarkets carry a growing range of legumes. You'll find them available dried or canned. With both kinds on hand, you're equipped to make dozens of flavourful dishes. Cook up a big batch of beans at a time and freeze them for future use. Caution: canned beans can have added salt. You may want to rinse them under cold running water.

There are three ways to prepare dried legumes for cooking. Always start by rinsing them well:

- Soak them overnight, adding 3 parts of water for 1 part beans. Discard soaking water before cooking.
- Add beans to water and bring to a boil. Let boil for 2 minutes, remove from heat and let stand for an hour. Discard soaking water before cooking.
- Combine beans and water in a microwaveable dish. Cover and microwave at full power for 15 minutes or until boiling. Let stand one hour. Drain.

Beans, beans, the musical fruit...
We all know about those unfortunate side effects. Soaking beans well and cooking them in fresh water will help to get rid of some of the sugars that produce gas.

Bean around the world?

Maybe the budget won't stretch to a trip to Europe or Mexico, but beans can take your tastebuds there. Legumes have been a part of diets worldwide for thousands of years. Even today, they are a dietary staple of billions. Think of Mexican tamales and bean burritos, Indian dahl, Middle Eastern hummus and falafel, Cuban black beans and rice, Italian minestrone soup, Chinese bean curd and bean sprouts—all dishes guaranteed to brighten up your dinner plate.

Compared with fresh beans or peas, dried varieties have more concentrated protein and other nutrients—enough, in fact, to grow a whole new plant.

The no-cook good news

You don't have to start from scratch. Good news if you're off to the store and supper has to be on the table in an hour. Use canned legumes instead. Black beans, white beans, red beans, lentils—you'll find them all on the shelf waiting to be packed in your cart and turned into something wonderful for supper. Just drain and rinse (to reduce any excess salt) and add to your favourite recipe.

Green, red, yellow or brown, lentils need no soaking. They take just 10 to 30 minutes to cook. Think of them as the express-lane legume.

fun food...fast
Bean salad

3 cups (750 mL) canned (or cooked) beans
1/2 cup each (125 mL) chopped green and red peppers and onion
1/4 cup (50 mL) low-calorie salad dressing

Toss together and enjoy.

What about soybeans?
Soy has been heralded as a "wonder food," but not all claims are grounded in science. Yes, research shows that soy may help prevent heart disease, but the evidence that soy prevents hormone-dependent cancers (breast cancer in women and prostate cancer in men), osteoporosis and menopausal symptoms is less clear.

What makes soybeans heart-healthy?
It is still unclear which substance in soy provides the heart-healthy benefits—it may be the high-quality protein, the phytochemicals (notably isoflavones) or even the fibre; plus, soy contains no cholesterol and is low in saturated fat.

How do I add soybeans to my diet?
Try soymilk as a beverage, tofu in a stir-fry, soynuts as a snack…You can find soy protein in veggie burgers, hot dogs and other meat substitutes. Sorry, soy sauce doesn't count.

Soybeans are different from other beans

- The only vegetable food that contains a complete protein
- Contains both soluble and insoluble fibre
- The only bean that contains fat. Soybean "fat" is mostly unsaturated.

A soybean feast

Soy doesn't just mean beans. It's the starting point for miso, soynuts, soy sauce, tempeh, tofu and TVP. Not sure which is which? Here's the scoop on soy products.

Miso   The term for a number of rich, salty condiments, indispensable to Japanese cooking. Store miso in the refrigerator and use sparingly because of its salt content.

Soynuts   Roasted whole soybeans. Look for the dry-roasted variety. These crunchy high-protein snacks are higher in fat if they have been oil-roasted.

Soy sauce   A mixture of soybeans, wheat flour and yeast that has been fermented for about 18 months. The liquid is extracted and then processed. Use sparingly because of its salt content.

Tempeh   Fermented soybeans make this traditional Indonesian food, which has a stronger flavour than tofu. You'll generally find it in the frozen foods case.

Tofu   A bland, soft, cheeselike food, tofu is made by curdling fresh hot soymilk with either nigari—a compound found in ocean water—or the compound calcium sulfate. The curds are then shaped and pressed into blocks. Because it's rich in protein and iron, the Chinese call it "meat without bones" and use it extensively in their cooking. Check the label. If the calcium salt has been used to curdle it, it's rich in calcium too.

    Tofu soaks up flavours like a sponge. It's easy and fast to prepare and easy to digest—and it doesn't cause gas! Firm tofu can replace meat in stir-fry dishes, soups or on the grill. It has more protein, calcium and fat than other forms of tofu. Try soft tofu in Asian soups.

    You'll find fresh tofu in the produce, dairy or deli sections. It's also sold as deep-fried strips and in pouches. You can buy fresh tofu in vacuum packs, in water-filled tubs or in aseptic brick packages. The packaged kind have a "best before" date. You can store the tofu varieties sealed in liquid. Once they are opened, drain off the water and replace water daily. Use within a week.

TVP (Textured Vegetable Protein)   When soy flour is compressed, its protein fibres change in structure and its texture becomes similar to ground beef. TVP is often used to extend products such as meats. It has a long shelf life because it is low in moisture.

Soy does not contain calcium, but soy beverages (used as milk alternatives) are often fortified with calcium. Check the calcium content in the Nutrition Facts table. Look at the fat and calorie content too. One cup soymilk has 1 tsp fat (the same as 2% milk but the fat is unsaturated). Lower-fat products are now available, so compare brands.

Edamame, the specialty soybean

Microwaved and tossed with coarse salt, edamame have become a popular snack food. These specialty soybeans, with fuzzy, dark green, plump pods, are picked when they're immature. You can eat them fresh but you'll usually find them frozen. Try them in salads, or as a snack or side dish. A healthy way to spend your fat budget, half a cup of edamame provides 125 calories and 1 tsp fat.

Nuts and seeds

Like legumes, nuts and seeds are crammed with nutrients. They *are* high in fat, but these are the right kind of heart-healthy unsaturated fats, and studies show that nut eaters may have a lower risk of heart disease. Nuts are also rich in minerals and vitamins, in particular vitamin E.

Agreed, eating nuts is a smart way to spend your fat budget, but use them sparingly. Try substituting them for protein sources higher in saturated fats, like meat and cheese. One ounce (1/4 cup or 30 g) chopped nuts provides roughly the same calories as 3 ounces (90 g) of lean meat.

Sprinkle nuts and seeds on salads and in stir-fries. As a snack they are a wiser choice than foods such as chips and chocolate bars, which are both high-fat and nutrient-deficient. But the fat in nuts and seeds adds up (see Fat Budget below), so if you are watching your weight, eat nuts one at a time rather than by the handful.

Nuts about nuts?

Here are some facts to munch on:
- One ounce of nuts (1/4 cup or 30 g chopped nuts) provides 165–200 calories and 3–4 tsp fat.
- Compared with other nuts, walnuts are highest in polyunsaturated fats; hazelnuts, pecans and pistachios are high in monounsaturated fats; almonds offer the most calcium and peanuts the most protein.

In a nutshell, enjoy a variety of nuts!

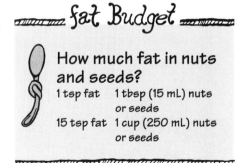

Fat Budget

How much fat in nuts and seeds?

1 tsp fat	1 tbsp (15 mL) nuts or seeds
15 tsp fat	1 cup (250 mL) nuts or seeds

Limit the number of roasted nuts you eat—they are often "fried" in coconut oil, a saturated fat, and may be heavily salted. Dry-roasted nuts are not cooked in oil but they contain almost as much fat.

Shell out for peanut butter

One, it's a good protein substitute. Two, it's a bargain. Peanut butter is peanuts ground into a paste. A staple in many homes, it's high in protein and that's why it's in the #2 part of your cart. It is rich in minerals and vitamin E but watch the fat content.

For variety, try butters made from other nuts, such as almonds. Look for them in specialty stores or in your supermarket.

Don't be misled by "light" peanut butter. It may be lower in fat, but chances are it has added sugar—and the same calories. Check the Nutrition Facts table on various brands and compare. My advice? Choose a regular peanut butter, enjoy the heart-healthy fat—and eat it in moderation.

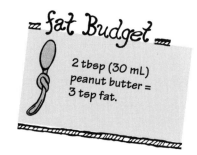

Fat Budget

2 tbsp (30 mL) peanut butter = 3 tsp fat.

• Making peanut butter sandwiches? You don't need to add butter or margarine.
• Don't be too concerned about a tiny amount of trans fat in regular peanut butter. It's there to stop the peanut butter from separating, and helps keep it fresh.
• Try "natural" peanut butter that contains only peanuts. To mix the oil that separates, turn the jar upside down in your pantry after you buy it, and then stir the oil into the peanut butter. Once opened, store it in the fridge. It stays mixed. Throw out a jar that has gone mouldy.

Meat and alternatives at a glance

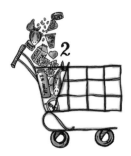

1. Choose lean cuts, trim visible fat and remove skin from poultry.
2. Choose fish more often.
3. Load up on beans, peas and lentils.
4. Enjoy nuts and nut butters—but use them sparingly.

Section **3** of your shopping cart

Fats, Oils and Others

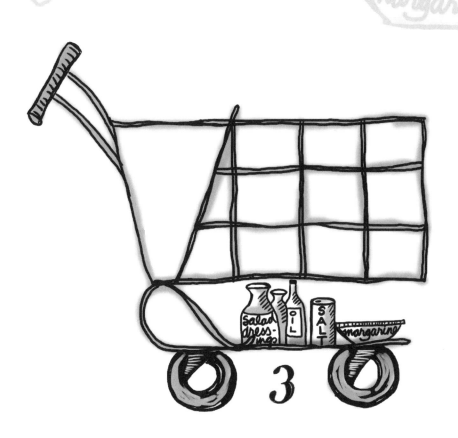

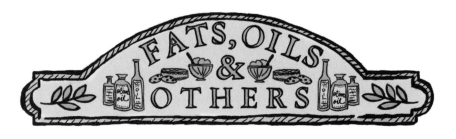

Think carefully about what you add to the #3 lower part of your cart. The less fat the better.

Now we get to the #3 part of your shopping cart—the other side of the nutrition rainbow. Be frugal here…seriously. You won't see these foods on the rainbow even though they're in Canada's Food Guide to Healthy Eating, because many of them offer too much fat relative to their nutritional value.

We're on the right track. Most of us make a real effort to cut back on animal fats, but that's only part of the story. Some fatty acids contribute to good health. Others may lead to disease. The secret is balance. Put healthy fats on your plate, by all means. But, at the same time, cut back on unhealthy saturated and trans fats.

Adding a fat, such as olive oil, to your diet for health reasons is great. But never forget, if the rest of your diet is still high in unhealthy fat, the added calories outweigh the health benefits.

So, live like a Mediterranean. Pump up your plate with the power of olives and olive oil. Reach for that canola oil, avocado and nuts. At the same time—and this is key—go lightly on butter and cream, and cut back on fried foods, baked goods and other foods processed with fats. That's why this part of your shopping cart calls for a very careful look. Fats, oils and others do fit—but choose wisely. Think lower. Think selectively. Think frugal.

Fat budgeting with fats and oils

Spend your fat budget wisely and choose healthier unsaturated fats more often. Or look for lower-fat versions. New ones are appearing every day.

Fat Budget

Fats, oils and others:

0	fat-free salad dressing
tsp fat	fat-free mayonnaise

1 tsp fat

1 tsp (5 mL) oil, cooking or salad*
1 tsp (5 mL) butter
1 tsp (5 mL) margarine
2 tsp (10 mL) low-fat margarine**
2 tsp (10 mL) nut butter*
1 tbsp (15 mL) low-fat mayonnaise
1 tbsp (15 mL) cream cheese
1 tbsp (15 mL) cheese spread
1 tbsp (15 mL) whipping cream
2 tbsp (30 mL) sour cream
2 tbsp (30 mL) half-and-half
2 tbsp (30 mL) shredded coconut

2 tsp fat

1 tbsp (15 mL) salad dressing*
1 tbsp (15 mL) mayonnaise
15 chips — potato, corn, nacho

3 tsp fat

1 small 50 g chocolate bar, plain

1 teaspoon fat = approximately 5 grams of fat.
These numbers are averages.
* Budget wisely—choose these healthier fats more often.
** Choose a non-hydrogenated margarine.

Health Check
™HEART AND STROKE FOUNDATION

Look for low-fat or
low-saturated-fat choices.

ALL STAR TIP

Try nut butters or non-hydrogenated margarine
instead of butter or
hydrogenated margarine.

Label Smarts

If the product you buy contains processed fat, look for
the words "non-hydrogenated fat" on the label. In the
Nutrition Facts table, the fat column should have
little if any trans fats.

We need to eat some fat

Fat plays an important role in overall nutrition.

- It carries the fat-soluble vitamins, A, D, E and K.
- It's a concentrated source of energy.
- It gives a glow to our skin and a shine to our hair.
- It helps us feel full by keeping food in the stomach longer.
- It provides the essential fatty acids that our bodies can't make and that
  we must get from foods.

1. Keeping your eye on visible fat

Some fats you can see, some you can't. Visible fat is the fat you can see, or the fat you buy to add to your food. Oils, margarines, butter, salad dressings, nuts, seeds, cream and coffee whiteners all come under this category.

Oils

The "oils" aisle is where you have the chance to spend your fat budget really wisely. But which is the best to choose from the ranks of bottles? Unfortunately, there's no one answer. All oils are a combination of fatty acids, and each fatty acid plays a different role. But some are better than others, so here are some guidelines to help you pick what's best for you.

Oil 101
Wondering which oil to use? Choose the one that's the lowest in saturated fat, has a good mixture of unsaturated fats, and is suited to your purpose, whether it's dressing a salad or baking a bran muffin.

Here are some healthy choices for oils:
• Low in saturated fat, the type of fat that raises LDL (the "bad" cholesterol): that means canola oil.
• High in monounsaturated fat, which lowers the LDL but not the HDL ("good" cholesterol): olive oil wins hands down, followed by canola oil. Olive oil is the primary source of fat in the Mediterranean diet, which is linked to a low incidence of heart disease. The vitamin E and phytochemicals it contains may also contribute to health.
• High in omega-3 fats: this type of polyunsaturated fat found in flaxseed, canola oil and soybean oil may help reduce your risk of heart disease.

Label Smarts
Look for this health claim on foods free of, or low in, saturated fats and trans fats: "A healthy diet low in saturated and trans fats may reduce the risk of heart disease."

DID YOU KNOW
Oils that are high in omega-3 fats are actually high in a fat called ALA (alpha-linolenic acid) that is converted by your body into omega-3 fats. It is more efficient to get your omega-3 fats from fatty fish.

Uncap the cooking magic of different oils

Use oils sparingly and in different ways. In my kitchen you'll find olive oil, which has a wonderful fruity flavour that is delicious on salads. Flaxseed oil works well on salads too. Canola oil is ideal when I need a cooking oil that has no taste. In the fridge is sesame oil, which has an intense nutty flavour— so I only need to use a little as a flavouring. Try it on stir-fries.

Cold-pressed, virgin, light—what do they mean?

Cold pressed means the oil was squeezed out of the olives by a mechanical press. No heat was used. The oil is rich-tasting and full, retaining much of the original olive flavour.

Extra virgin or **virgin** refers to the difference in acid content, not the fat. Oil from the first pressing is often called "extra virgin" and is the most delicate in flavour. Virgin olive oil comes from the second pressing.

Light olive oil describes a lighter colour, fragrance or texture. It does not refer to "light" in fat or calories.

All oils are 100% fat.

I'm new to flaxseed oil. Any tips?

Flaxseed oil, also called linseed oil, has a pleasant, nutty taste. Although it isn't an all-purpose oil (you can't use it for sautéing or frying), it is delicious used cold in, for instance, salad dressings. It is expensive and it spoils easily (the dark bottle it's sold in extends its shelf life), so buy it in small quantities and keep it in the fridge.

Flaxseeds contain the heart-healthy soluble fibre found in oats. Sprinkle ground flaxseeds on cereals, salads or cooked veggies. Buy the seeds pre-ground for convenience, or grind them just before use to preserve their flavour and nutrition. Store ground flaxseeds in the fridge.

How to add less oil to your food

- When you're cooking with oil, try to use nonstick pans and heat the oil before you add the food. That way, the food sits in the oil for a shorter time and absorbs less.

- Using mellow balsamic or fruit vinegars in salad dressings lets you use less oil. Mustard, herbs and garlic will also boost the flavour.

- Spray your baking pans with a cooking spray that contains vegetable oil (such as corn or soy) plus lecithin, which helps oil and water solutions stick together. These sprays prevent sticking by forming a thin film between the food and the baking tray. Shake the can well before using and use only on cold surfaces.

- Make your own oil spray by filling a spray bottle with your favourite oil. Just pump and spray. If you use a see-through bottle, you will be amazed to see how little oil you actually need to coat a pan or spray your salad greens.

"No cholesterol" does not mean that the oil is special. All oils are vegetable products, so they don't contain cholesterol anyway. Manufacturers could just as well put "no diamond dust" on the label.

The name "canola" comes from <u>CAN</u>adian <u>O</u>il, <u>L</u>ow <u>A</u>cid. Canola oil is also called rapeseed oil.

Margarine and butter

What's the wiser spread for your bread? Both have the same total fat content and therefore the same number of calories, but...

Butter contains cholesterol—it comes from an animal source. Margarine is cholesterol-free—it's made from vegetable oils, a plant source.

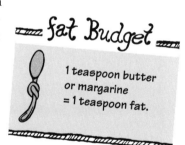

Fat Budget

1 teaspoon butter or margarine = 1 teaspoon fat.

Both hydrogenated margarine and butter are high in saturated fat. What's more, during processing some of the fat in hydrogenated margarine turns into trans fatty acids. Both of these fats tend to raise cholesterol.

The wiser choice for heart health? Non-hydrogenated margarine. It has no cholesterol or trans fats and is low in saturated fat.

Watching your weight? The less of either spread you use, the better.

Instead of spreading butter or margarine on your bread, adopt the Mediterranean habit of dipping it in a swirl of olive oil and balsamic vinegar.

For your health's sake, choose a margarine that is non-hydrogenated. The Nutrition Facts table should list almost no trans fats and hardly any saturated fat.

Looking for a lower-fat/lower-calorie margarine? Containing at least half the fat and calories of regular margarines, "light" margarines usually fit the bill. Check the Nutrition Facts table. Their water content makes them unsuitable for cooking—and they can make toast soggy—but they're ideal for sandwiches or with baked or mashed potatoes.

Palm oil added in small amounts to non-hydrogenated margarine makes the margarine spreadable without creating trans fats.

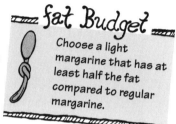

fat Budget

Choose a light margarine that has at least half the fat compared to regular margarine.

Cream cheese lovers, rejoice

Compared to butter or margarine, cream cheese has one-third as much fat so it's a good choice—provided you don't use three times as much! You'll find some wonderful tasty new choices on the market flavoured with smoked salmon, garlic or fruit. Look for new lower-fat cream cheeses that have about half the fat. No, you can't count it as a milk serving.

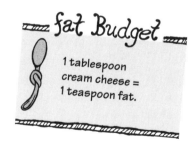

fat Budget

1 tablespoon cream cheese = 1 teaspoon fat.

Salad dressings and mayonnaise

Most of us are looking for lower-fat products, and manufacturers have responded. Browse the shelves and you'll come upon lots of low-fat or fat-free salad dressing and mayonnaise. Check the label to find out how many grams of fat each one contains—and zero in on the one with the least.

Label Smarts

If it says "low calorie" on the label, a salad dressing is low-fat too. The calories in a dressing come mostly from fat.

ALL STAR TIP

- Make the lunchtime sandwich a variety show. Try other spreads such as salsa, mustard, chutney, cranberry sauce, ketchup or relish. If you're using mayonnaise, skip the margarine or butter.
- Checked the vinegar section recently? What a choice! Red wine, white wine and herb-flavoured vinegars. Balsamic and apple cider vinegar. Raspberry and strawberry vinegar. All waiting to add impact to salads, sauces—even desserts. Make your own in the summer months when berries are ripe and fresh herbs are plentiful.

For flavour's sake, be a little saucy

Borrow ideas from other cuisines around the world and use high-powered sauces for instant flavour. Try teriyaki, hoisin, plum and fiery chili sauce from Asia. Experiment with Mexican salsa or British Worcestershire sauce. Although they're low in fat, some of these sauces may be higher in salt. Use just a touch—that's all you need.

fun food...fast
Dazzling dressings

Creamy Homemade Dressings
Be creative! Blend low-fat yogurt or soft yogurt cheese with a little low-fat mayonnaise. Season with fresh herbs, a minced clove of garlic, fresh basil, dill, oregano, black pepper or chili powder.

Great Vinaigrette Varieties
Mix 2 parts oil—or try even less (see below)—with 1 part vinegar and your favourite herbs. For variety, try red wine vinegar, rice vinegar, balsamic vinegar or raspberry vinegar.

Balsamic Orange Vinaigrette
1/3 cup (75 mL) orange juice
2 tbsp (30 mL) balsamic vinegar
2 tbsp (30 mL) olive oil
1 tsp (5 mL) dry mustard
1/4 cup (50 mL) water
2 tsp (10 mL) chopped parsley
Combine and whisk. Refrigerate for a few hours. Serve with mild-flavoured greens—25 calories and 2 grams fat per 1 tbsp serving.

Keep an eye on your salt intake!

ALL STAR TIP

Salt is the most commonly used seasoning, and most of us eat too much of it. On top of what you shake on your food, salt is added to processed foods, snack foods and fast foods.

We are not all salt sensitive. Adding salt to your diet does not mean that you will develop high blood pressure. But it seems wise to cut back on sodium whenever possible. Salt is a taste you get used to; use less of it, and you may be surprised at how flavourful food is.

Don't rely on salt for flavour. Here are some easy ways to cut down.

• Be aware of the salt you add when you're cooking and eating. Try taping over half the holes in the salt shaker.

• Use more fresh foods such as homemade soups rather than canned.

• Try spices and seasonings instead of salt. Lemon, mustard powder, garlic, ginger, curry, thyme, parsley or paprika can all lift a dish from bland to mind-blowing.

• Making your own stock and bouillon will let you cut down on the salt.

• Read labels on processed foods and choose low-salt products whenever possible.

• If you're using a salt substitute, check with your doctor.

Q&A

Sea salt or table salt: any difference?

Although unrefined sea salt may contain small amounts of some minerals, once refined it's almost the same as ordinary salt, but without the benefit of being iodized.

DID YOU KNOW?

A little DASH'll do ya. According to a well-regarded anti-hypertensive diet called Dietary Approaches to Stop Hypertension, or DASH, the ideal diet for lowering blood pressure is loaded with fruits, veggies and low-fat dairy products. Cutting salt and caffeine is only part of the plan.

The Nutrition Facts table lists the percentage of daily value for sodium. Compare products and, in general, pick the one with the least sodium. As a reference, 1 teaspoon of salt contains almost 2,400 mg sodium. You need no more than that in a day. You may be surprised how much sodium there is in your favourite foods.

Here's what a lower sodium claim means:

Sodium-free	less than 5 mg
Low in sodium	140 mg or less
Reduced or lower in sodium	at least 25% less
No added sodium	none added during processing
Lightly salted	at least 50% less

Cream—sweet or sour, it's sinful

There's something unique about the flavour and silkiness of cream. Too bad it's high in fat. See how it fits into your fat budget before you indulge.

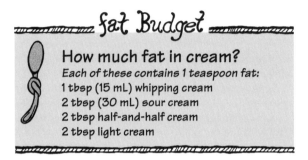

Fat Budget

How much fat in cream?
Each of these contains 1 teaspoon fat:
1 tbsp (15 mL) whipping cream
2 tbsp (30 mL) sour cream
2 tbsp half-and-half cream
2 tbsp light cream

Here's the HeartSmart™ way to give coffee a stir

Use low-fat milk instead of cream, and skim milk powder instead of coffee whitener.

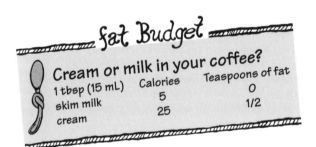

DID YOU KNOW
Non-dairy coffee whiteners may be cholesterol free but they're not fat free. Often the vegetable oil is hydrogenated or the oil used is palm or coconut oil—high in saturated fat. Many brands have more calories per serving than light cream. A far better buy is skim milk powder.

ALL STAR TIP

When a recipe calls for sour cream, use low-fat or nonfat versions, or try low-fat yogurt cheese instead. See page 88.

Fat Budget

Cream or milk in your coffee?

1 tbsp (15 mL)	Calories	Teaspoons of fat
skim milk	5	0
cream	25	1/2

2. Watch out for invisible fat

Snack foods can hide fat—often too much and often saturated. Cut back on high-fat processed foods. Go slow as you add these to the #3 part of your cart.

Processed foods are often high in unhealthy trans fats. Read labels. Check the Nutrition Facts table and choose products with the least fat overall, and the least saturated and trans fat per serving.

HeartSmart Tip Snack counterattack

- Keep your fridge stocked with fresh veggies and fruit for quick and delicious low-fat snacks.
- Buy lower-fat snacks such as plain popcorn and rice cakes rather than chips or high-fat cookies.
- Choose sherbet, low-fat frozen yogurt or low-fat dairy desserts more often than ice cream.
- Choose cookies and crackers with less than 1 teaspoon fat per serving. More ideas? See Simple Snacks, page 130.

Potato chips, corn chips, tortilla chips, cheese puffs

In themselves, potatoes and corn are low-fat foods. Fry them in oil to make chips and look what happens. Suddenly just a few chips—about 15—add up to 2 teaspoons (10 g) of fat. Not to mention the added salt. Heavy on the fat budget.

- Keep your eyes open for baked chips that are lower in fat and salt. But be careful. Watching your weight? They are not much lower in calories. The temptation is to eat more. Check the Nutrition Facts table for calories—and check the serving size. You may be unpleasantly surprised! In a Mexican mood? Serve baked tortilla chips with low-fat salsa rather than high-fat guacamole.
- "Low in saturated fat" on a label doesn't necessarily mean that a snack is low in total fat. Don't be misled and think you can eat more.

Popcorn

Granted, it's simple to make, but packaged microwave popcorn is high in fat. Look for the low-fat varieties. A better idea? Make your own popcorn on top of the stove using minimal oil, or use a hot air popper, and salt sparingly.

Picking microwave popcorn? Read the Nutrition Facts table and choose popcorn with less than 60 calories for 3 cups popped.

For the Love of Chocolate

DID YOU KNOW

Chocolate consumption is on the rise, perhaps because eating chocolate releases serotonin, a brain chemical that makes us feel good. Or maybe it is the amines that increase your heart rate? The caffeine that gives you a mental boost? Or just that yummy melt-in-your-mouth experience? Choose the best chocolate you can afford. The lower-quality stuff is made from saturated oils (such as palm and coconut oil) whereas high-quality dark chocolate contains flavonoids, the phytochemicals found also in tea, that may help to reduce the risk of heart disease and certain cancers.

The reality check: chocolate is not a drug, a medicine or (sadly) a food group. It is still candy. A typical small chocolate bar (50 g) contains roughly 270 calories, 2 to 3 teaspoons fat and loads of sugar. Remember, 1 teaspoon fat = approximately 5 grams fat. When your craving overwhelms you, choose the smallest amount of the highest-quality dark chocolate...and enjoy!

ALL STAR TIP

- Carob flour is low in fat, but it is combined with coconut oil or hydrogenated vegetable oil for use in chocolate bars so the fat content is as high as chocolate. Whichever way you cut it, carob or chocolate takes big bites out of your fat budget.
- Dry chocolate-milk powder mixed with skim or 1% milk is a good, lower-fat way to feed that chocolate craving.

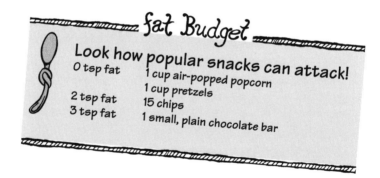

Fat Budget

Look how popular snacks can attack!

0 tsp fat	1 cup air-popped popcorn
	1 cup pretzels
2 tsp fat	15 chips
3 tsp fat	1 small, plain chocolate bar

Fats, oils and others at a glance

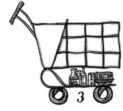

1. Reduce the total quantity of fat in your diet.
2. Think quality. Choose unsaturated fats.
3. Take control of how you spend your fat budget.

Mighty Meals
Mighty Quick

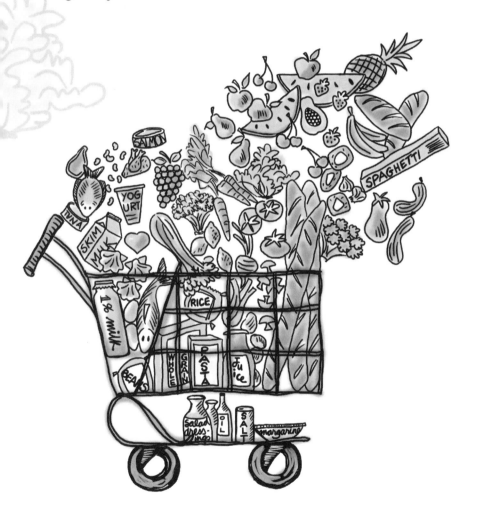

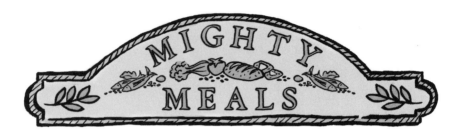

MIGHTY MEALS

Fill your plate the same way you fill your HeartSmart™ shopping cart. Load up with grains, fruit and veggies, choose lower-fat meat and milk products, and go slow on the fats and oils.

Because I'm a dietitian, people often ask me, "What do you feed your family? Do you ponder over cookbooks all the time? Do you spend hours cooking up a storm?"

To be honest, I have shelves full of tempting books. I love to read them and yes, I love to cook. But I usually only try new recipes when we're entertaining. Sound familiar? On a daily basis, I want no-brainer dishes that are quick, simple, tasty and nutritious. Meals that are mighty in nutrition, that I can make from memory—and that are mighty quick.

We need three meals a day and nutritious snacks. And the better balanced they are, the easier it is to stay well, maintain a healthy weight and control our fat budgets. Breakfast is usually fast and functional. Lunch can be at home or in lunch bags packed with savvy and skill. Supper is loaded with nutrition, and made in minutes.

How to have Mighty Meals every day

These days not many of us have time to follow formal recipes on a daily basis. We need to work with ideas—concepts. These are mine.

As I've shown you throughout this book, fat and nutrient intake are better managed over several days than on a recipe-by-recipe basis. Just follow the concepts and rest assured, they all add up to HeartSmart nutrition.

Beginning with **breakfast**

The most important meal of the day. Your body hasn't had nourishment in many hours. Your day lies ahead. No wonder you need refuelling. I start every day with a fresh fruit, maybe an orange or a banana, a large bowl of cereal (made from a mix of three different high-fibre cereals) with skim milk and a cup of tea. Fruit, grains and milk—already I've had servings from three of the four bands of the Canada's Food Guide rainbow, and I've chosen a variety of foods from the #1 part of my shopping cart and a lower-fat choice from #2.

One-minute Mighty **breakfasts**

All of these are nutritious, delicious, low fat—and fast to make. Choose whole-grain breads (bread, bagels, English muffins) whenever possible.

"Toasted" Cottage Cheese
Spread low-fat cottage cheese on an English muffin. Sprinkle with a mixture of cinnamon and sugar. Top with sliced bananas or raisins. Broil in toaster oven.

Super Slices
Bagels or whole-wheat toast spread with low-fat cream cheese or peanut butter and jam.

Microwaved Eggs
Mix up 2 beaten eggs in a mug (one whole and one egg white is a lower-fat option). Microwave for 40 seconds at full power and serve with toast.

Power Blender Shake
Blend one cup low-fat milk, a banana, 1 tsp (5 mL) of vanilla and 1 tbsp (15 mL) of honey until frothy. Yum! Other days, add a tablespoon of peanut butter or a 1/2 cup (125 mL) of fruit-flavoured low-fat yogurt or fresh fruit.

Two-Minute Lower-cholesterol French Toast (worth that extra minute)
Whisk together 2 egg whites, 2 whole eggs, 1/4 cup (50 mL) low-fat milk, a few drops of vanilla, 2 tsp (10 mL) of sugar and a pinch of cinnamon. One by one, dip 8 slices of bread into the mixture, coating them well. Lightly grease a nonstick pan and brown each slice on both sides. Makes enough for 4.

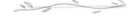

Power lunch bags

By the middle of the day many of us are out of the house. It's all too easy to head for the closest fast-food joint—and possibly blow our fat budget and our pocketbook for the day. We may even skip lunch. Packing a healthy lunch bag is easy once you get into the habit, and it's far better nutritionally.

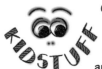

Our kids spend half their weekday at school. What is your child eating? Kids need food for energy, to grow and to help them concentrate—but it's got to be healthy food. Poor choices are leading more and more kids to obesity and diabetes. School lunches are a great way to teach them good habits. What are the options?

1. The school cafeteria. One of my personal pet peeves is the lunches offered in so many high schools. Choices are limited, and the foods can be loaded with fat and refined carbohydrates. As a parent, lobby for better food for your kids.

2. The corner store or fast-food outlet. Most offer the least-nutritious choices. Hot dogs, nachos and iced tea. Cheeseburger, fries and a large pop. Fat, salt and sugar. Yuck.

3. They make their own. Absolutely, teach your kids to be responsible for making their own lunch, but see that it's nutritious (usually the last thing on their minds, especially busy teens).

4. You make lunch for them. Yes, I made school lunches with, or for, both my kids until the day they finished high school. That's 4,800 lunches (200 lunches per year for 12 years), but the time and commitment were more than worth it. You're teaching them, subtly, that you value their health, that eating well makes a difference and that the effort is worth it. Send them with homemade lunches if you possibly can. Actions speak louder than words.

Mighty lunch bag shopping list

Pack a lunch the same way you fill your HeartSmart shopping cart. Load up with whole grains, fruits and veggies. Choose lean meat and low-fat milk products. Be creative with legumes. Go light on the fat you add. Picture a 1-2-3 lunch bag, just like your shopping cart.

30 minutes of organization = 1-minute lunches

• Tasty sandwich fillings. High-powered fruits and veggies. If you've got them all at hand, you'll use them. A system like this saves you time and money. You just have to be "dedicated."

• DEDICATE one KITCHEN DRAWER for lunch supplies. Here's what goes in it: paper or reusable nylon bags, thermoses, assorted microwaveable plastic containers, drinking bottles, plastic utensils and napkins, a notepad and pen so you can write a quick few lines. Finding a note that says "I love you," or "Hope that exam goes well," will brighten anyone's afternoon.

• DEDICATE one part of the FRIDGE for lunch-only items: yogurt, milk, juice, sandwich fixings (not just the fillings but the mustard and the low-fat mayo). Let your family know that it's hands off for casual snacking.

Build a super sandwich

The Bread

Whole-grain bread, bagels, pitas, buns, submarines, Kaiser buns, dinner rolls or English muffins.

The Spread

A smear, no more, of margarine or butter or mayonnaise (choose the low-fat or fat-free varieties). Mustard, salsa, chutney, cranberry sauce or relish to boost flavour.

The Fillers

Lots of lettuce, tomato, cucumber, onions—even sliced oranges. Whatever you have, load up. Layer wet things like tomato between two other fillers and the bread won't go soggy.

The Filling

Lean meats such as turkey breast, low-fat ham or lean beef. Canned salmon or tuna (be light on what you moisten it with). Peanut butter. Chopped hard-cooked egg.

Wrap and Roll

Building a wrap or roll is the same as building a sandwich—and the same principles apply for the spread, the fillers and the filling.

Try these on a tortilla:
- Spread with mango chutney, and top with roasted lean chicken, leftover seasoned rice and chopped cilantro.
- Spread with light cream cheese, and fill with smashed chickpeas, roasted red pepper and salad fixings.
- Spread with honey mustard, and layer with a slice of ham, tomatoes and lettuce.
- Spread with low-fat mayonnaise, flaked tuna, green onions, shredded carrots and lettuce.

Plan leftovers for lunch

The lunchroom microwave opens the door to variety. HeartSmart pasta dishes, rice and vegetables, soups and stews can warm you up the next day or can be frozen in lunch-sized portions to make a welcome return appearance later on.

Substantial salads made with beans, grains or pasta also hold up well and make a nice change from sandwiches. So make lots, and make lunch even easier.

Fending off those sneaky snack attacks

Snacking is a national pastime. We all do it. Kids do it whenever they can. Teens do it constantly. But…if you keep the fridge and the pantry filled with tasty foods that are low in fat, snacks can be a way to boost everyone's nutrition.

Put fruit juice on your shopping list instead of soft drinks. Keep tubs of yogurt and yogurt-cheese dips in the fridge and a platter of crisp cut-up vegetables right beside them. Buy whole-grain breads and crackers, and low-fat cheese instead of cookies and chips.

Mighty simple snacks

- Low-fat milk, cheese or yogurt
- Cereal
- Fresh fruit
- Bagels or pita bread spread thinly with light cream cheese
- Cut veggies prebagged so that they're user-friendly. Serve with low-fat or fat-free salad dressing or low-fat yogurt-cheese dips
- Homemade low-fat muffins
- Mini-pizza on English muffin or pita bread
- Low-fat cheese and crackers
- Unbuttered popcorn—air popped is best. Keep the air-popper on your kitchen counter so it's easy to use. Toss with herbs or spices.
- Low-fat yogurt—look for 1% milk fat or less and mix with cut-up fruit
- Vegetable or tomato juice
- Unsweetened ready-to-eat cereal
- Fruit kebabs—just thread whole strawberries, grapes, banana pieces or orange segments on wooden skewers
- Rice cakes spread thinly with peanut butter, almond butter or light cream cheese
- Frozen juice popsicles or light fudgsicles
- Hummus and pita bread
- Homemade corn chips. Cut tortillas into wedges. Bake in single layer at 400°F (200°C) for 8 minutes, or until lightly browned and crisp (or, make your own bagel chips by toasting sliced-up bagels in the oven and dip in salsa).

DID YOU KNOW

Guess how much sugar there is in a can of pop. A teaspoon? Two? Guess again. A glass of pop contains 7.5 teaspoons of sugar. It's like eating a handful of sugar cubes.

Fruit drink isn't the same as fruit juice. If it doesn't say "juice" on the bottle or package, then it isn't. There may be as little as 10% juice in fruit punch, cocktail or beverage. Your best bet is to buy products labelled "juice" or you may be paying a premium for expensive sugar water! Remember, the ingredient at the top of the list is present in the greatest quantity.

Have a cuppa...tea or coffee

• Despite scores of studies on caffeine, no conclusive evidence suggests that it is harmful. According to Nutrition Recommendations for Canadians, a moderate caffeine intake is 4 cups a day of drip coffee. (Check the size of your coffee cup—some of the new cups can be as large as two regular cups.) Tea, chocolate, colas and some over-the-counter medications also contain caffeine.

• A low-fat latte makes a tasty snack, but watch the fat and calories in your favourite specialty coffee (see page 84).

• Limit caffeine if you have high blood pressure or your doctor has advised you to relieve symptoms of gastric distress.

• Green tea is a popular choice these days, but feel free to sip any cuppa you like. Green, black and red (oolong) tea all come from the leaf of the *Camellia sinensis*. They contain phytochemicals called flavonoids, and there is mounting evidence that they act as antioxidants in a test tube (see antioxidants on page 61). But the jury is still out on their effect in your body.

Dinners in a dash

Fill your plate the same way you fill your HeartSmart shopping cart. Be lavish with grains and vegetables. Use meat as an accent. Go slow on the fats and oils. Make the main event a delicious stir-fry, pasta, or soup and salad. Read about the Power of the Plate (page 12).

Remember the old saying: "Eat breakfast like a king, lunch like a queen and dinner like a pauper." The last meal of the day can be a lot lighter than we're used to.

Add up all the variations you can create around a few favourites, and you could put a different dinner on the table every night of the year. What's even better? These mighty dishes are so simple they don't even need recipes. Just remember a few easy steps.

Low in fat, high in flavour: six quick tips

Fat carries flavours, which is why we sometimes find it hard to cut back. The trick? Replace it with other intense and satisfying flavours—or let a food's own great, natural taste shine through.

Here's how:

1. Cook rice, beans and grains in stock with added herbs and garlic.
2. Add zest and shine to grilled foods with mustards, jams and chutneys.
3. Use nonstick cookware so you need less cooking fat.
4. Replace oil with stock, juice or wine to moisten and baste meats.
5. Use a spray bottle filled with oil to lightly dress a salad or to spritz your wok, pan or baking tray.
6. Add herbs and spices. They're terrific flavour boosters that let you limit fat and salt. Feel free to experiment.

Kids do what you do, not what you say.
Have your kids compare the size of their own palm and fist to the food on their plate. It's a simple, nag-free way to talk about nutrition, serving size and healthy food choices.

Watching your weight? Here's the way to fill your plate:
MEATS: One serving should be the size and thickness of your palm. This means more for the average man than the average woman.
GRAINS OR STARCHY CARBOHYDRATES: One portion is roughly the size of your fist.
SALADS AND VEGGIES: Half your plate, or more, should be vegetables. Super-size them.
FATS: Less is better. Spend your fat budget on health-giving unsaturated fats.
Still hungry? Load up with salads and veggies.

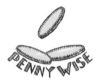

Got a sunny window in your kitchen? It's the perfect spot for a few containers of fresh herbs. That way you'll get used to snipping them to add to soups and savoury dishes—with sparkling results. Fresh basil with tomatoes is a magical combination. Oregano or savory really wake up green beans. French and Italian herbs—rosemary, thyme, marjoram and sage—all add flair to pastas, vegetables and casseroles.

• Ground spices lose their flavour quickly. Buy a little at a time—or buy them whole and grind as needed. Store them in a cool, dry place.

• Before you add fresh herbs to a dish, rub them between your hands to release their flavour.

• Increase the flavour of spices (but not dried herbs) by heating them in a dry pan until just fragrant.

What about frozen dinners?

They're convenient, yes, but often not a nutritious choice. Read the labels before you add them to your shopping cart. Look for lean entrées and meats that are lower in fat and calories. Remember, the ingredients at the top of the list are there in the greatest quantity.

Fat: look for dinners with less than 30% calories from fat.

Salt: look for products with as little as possible. You can always bump up flavour by adding lemon juice or herbs.

Make your own frozen TV dinners. Buy compartmentalized freezable, microwaveable containers and use them for leftovers—planned or unplanned.

Stir-fry suppers

Stir-fries are a deceptively simple way to create a host of different dishes, to make the most of a little meat and to enjoy a bounty of tender-crisp vegetables.

Stir-fry suppers

Preheat your wok or nonstick pan. Spray or add a smidgen of oil and swirl around to coat the surface. You'll need less oil provided it's hot enough when you cook the veggies. Even better, use stock or try low-fat salad dressings. Add chopped garlic and ginger and stir-fry for a few seconds.

Introduce the meat and alternatives group: sliced lean beef, chunks of chicken breast, tofu or scallops. Stir-fry these before you cook the vegetables. Keep warm on a plate, then add when vegetables are tender.

Add veggies—cut them ahead of time (or use up those snacking vegetables that have been in the fridge for a day or two). Start with those that take longest to cook such as onions, broccoli or cauliflower. End with snow peas or mushrooms that cook in a wink. My favourite combo bursts with colour and texture: mushrooms, broccoli, red and green pepper, chickpeas, zucchini, canned baby corn. Make the palette on your plate a delight to your palate.

Wake up your tastebuds with something different. Add chunks of pineapple or apple.

Push stir-fried ingredients to sides of wok or frying pan and add zing to your stir-fry with sauce. Cook until thickened. Here are some of my favourites.

Basic Sauce

2 tsp (10 mL) cornstarch   1 tbsp (15 mL) water
1/2 cup (125 mL) stock   2 tsp (10 mL) light soy sauce
2 tsp (10 mL) honey   1/4 tsp (1 mL) garlic powder
Mix cornstarch with water until smooth. Add other ingredients.

Variations

- SWEET AND SOUR: use pineapple juice instead of chicken stock—a bonus, it's lower in salt. Toss in some pineapple pieces and stir-fry. Yum.

- SZECHUAN SPICY SAUCE: use chili oil in place of cooking oil and add a pinch of dried chili peppers to the basic sauce.

- THAI SAUCE: add 2 tbsp (30 mL) hoisin sauce, 2 tsp (10 mL) each of sesame oil and rice vinegar and 1 tsp (5 mL) dry mustard instead of the soy sauce and honey.

Sprinkle a few toasted peanuts, cashews, sesame seeds or almonds over your stir-fry. Go lightly, these contain fat. Serve with cooked rice (see page 50).

Super chicken

You can't beat chicken for versatility. Choose breasts, remove the skin and go dipping for flavour.

Amazin' chicken dippin'

Remove skin from chicken breasts. Allow one half per person. Season it sensationally. Combine and pour over chicken one of the following:
- Equal amounts of low-fat Italian or Russian dressing mixed with plum or apricot jam. Onion soup mix contributes a wonderful flavour but it does add salt.
- 2 tbsp (30 mL) each Worcestershire sauce, vinegar and chutney, 2 1/2 tbsp (35 mL) ketchup and a chopped green onion, mixed and marinated for 30 minutes.
- 1/4 cup lemon juice, 2 tsp (10 mL) oil, 2 tsp (10 mL) prepared mustard, mixed and marinated.
  Or spread chicken generously with Dijon mustard and toss in bag of breadcrumbs until coated. Amazingly simple. Outstandingly good.

Bake uncovered at 350°F (180°C) for one hour.
  Serve with low-fat french "fries" (page 71) cooked alongside, and a stir-fry of zucchini and tomatoes seasoned with basil, garlic and parsley. Check out Veggie power (page 69). Green salad on the side.

Fish made fabulous

Plain, simple fish is the perfect low-fat choice for a healthy meal. Bake, broil or grill, adding flavour with herbs, citrus juice or spicy salsas.

Wash white fish such as cod, halibut or sole. Pat dry with a paper towel and place in a single layer in a lightly greased casserole.

A world of fish

- Go Mexican and cover with salsa—Spanish for "sauce."
- For Chinese seasoning add fresh ginger, lower-salt soy sauce and scallions.
- Enjoy Japanese teriyaki by marinating in a mixture of 2 tbsp (30 mL) Dijon mustard, 3 tbsp (45 mL) brown sugar, 2 tbsp (30 mL) lower-salt soy sauce, 1 tsp (5 mL) sesame oil and 1 tsp (5 mL) sesame seeds. A sensation.
- Marinate fish for 10 minutes in a commercial marinade or your own made from a finely chopped tomato and red pepper, 1 tbsp (15 mL) each of olive oil and balsamic vinegar and a big pinch of basil, either dried or fresh.
- Pour a can of creamed, low-salt canned soup (mushroom or celery) over the fish.

Add chopped or sliced vegetables and bake uncovered at 350°F (180°C) —or bake the fish on top of the veggies and baste frequently. Bake fish 10 minutes for every inch of thickness.

Serve with rice (page 50), pasta or potatoes and a green salad.

Low-fat Breaded Fish Sticks

Go double dipping with filleted strips of fish:

- Dip in a mixture of low-fat milk and egg white.
- Then dip in dry breadcrumbs seasoned with thyme, basil or dill.
- Line baking sheet with foil, spray with nonstick cooking spray and layer with fish sticks. Bake at 400°F (210°C) for 10 minutes.

Meat marvels

Switch gears on meat—consider it an accent rather than the main course. Choose lean meat, trim external fat and marinate to tenderize.

Meat that s-t-r-e-t-c-h-e-s

Remember, a serving is the size of the palm of your hand. Make your meat s-t-r-e-t-c-h. Here's how.

Kebabs
Alternate cubes of marinated lean meat or poultry with cubed green peppers, whole cherry tomatoes, mushrooms and pineapple pieces or apricot halves. Broil or grill 3–5 minutes each side. Serve with rice and a large salad.

Fajitas
In nonstick frying pan or wok, sauté lean meat in 2 tsp oil or stock until cooked. Set aside. Sauté onions and peppers until tender. Add meat and heat through. Season to taste. Spread hoisin sauce on warmed flour tortillas (wrap in foil and heat at 350°F [180°C] for about 8 minutes), cover with meat and vegetable mixture, shredded lettuce and diced tomato. Roll and enjoy.

Let your family create their personalized fajitas—try roasted vegetables, salsa or non-fat yogurt as toppings, pita bread instead of tortillas, and chicken in place of meat.

Stir-fries
Add thinly sliced meat to your mound of vegetables. Serve on a bed of rice or pasta.

M-m-m-marinades
Lean meat doesn't have to be tough and dry. Marinating it for 4 to 8 hours in wine or vinegar will make it meltingly tender and flavourful. Here's my favourite:

Chop an onion, mince a garlic clove and grate a chunk of fresh ginger. Add 2 tbsp (30 mL) each of brown sugar, lemon juice, ketchup, Worcestershire sauce and oil and mix in 1/2 cup (125 mL) lower-salt soy sauce. Marinate lean meat overnight in the mixture. Barbecue or grill for 3 to 5 minutes on each side. Slice thinly on the diagonal.

Pasta power

Long skinny spaghetti, linguine and fettuccini. Spirals, shells and pasta shaped like little ears. You'll find at least one for every day of the month!

Pasta is a staple in many homes—but go easy. Standard pasta is a refined carbohydrate and it is tempting to eat too much, especially if you are watching your weight. Tips to make it fit your nutrition plan:

• Choose whole-wheat pasta.

• Remember the power of the plate. Use less pasta, load up your low-fat sauce with veggies, and add lean protein. Skip the garlic bread and have salad instead.

Add pasta to a big pot of boiling water—skip the salt. Boil dried pasta uncovered, stirring occasionally, until tender but firm, about 12 minutes. Drain immediately in colander (there's no need to rinse), toss with sauce and serve.

Sensationally simple quick tomato sauce

Sauté chopped onion and garlic in broth or a teaspoon of olive oil. Add a can of plum tomatoes (break them up with a wooden spoon). Simmer for 30 minutes. Add dried or fresh basil and season to taste. Hint: make lots and freeze the leftovers, or use a ready-made tomato-based sauce. Add chopped fresh vegetables such as peppers, mushrooms or zucchini. Throw in a handful of frozen peas—or any other frozen vegetable. Stir in a drained can of tuna, add scallops for a special treat, or leftover cubed chicken can go in at the last minute so it just warms through.

Top the pasta with sauce, parmesan cheese and freshly ground pepper. Serve with salad.

Match pasta shapes to pasta sauces

• Hollow pastas (elbows, shells, rigatoni): let them trap thick, chunky sauces.
• Wide pasta (fettuccini): mix with creamy sauces.
• Long pastas (spaghetti, linguine): dress them up with tomato or seafood sauces.
• Small pasta shapes (orzo and alphabet noodles): use in soups.
• Fresh pasta: try light tomato-based sauces—fresh absorbs more liquid than dried pasta.

One tablespoon (15 mL) of grated parmesan has only 2 grams fat and 25 calories, but it is fairly high in sodium.

Souper soups

Shout it out…this is one of the best-kept nutrition secrets in town. Soup can be low in calories, high in fibre and loaded with nutrients. Want some examples?

Please sir—may I have some more?

Chicken Soup to Build On
Best the next day—it's worth the wait.

Cover raw chicken parts with 16 cups (4 L) of cold water. Use breasts if you want to eat the chicken, economical backs and necks if you just want the flavour. Bring to a boil and skim. Add sliced vegetables—onions, carrots, celery stalks with their leaves, a skinned tomato and a parsnip. Season with 1/2 tsp (2 mL) thyme, 1 bay leaf, 4 cloves garlic, 6 peppercorns, salt and pepper to taste. Simmer for about 2 hours. Place in fridge overnight and remove the fat that settles on the top.

Make enough soup and you can enjoy it several ways: enjoy as is; add noodles, macaroni or rice; or strain and concentrate to make a handy chicken stock for cooking.

Serve with whole-grain buns and a green salad. Fresh fruit is a nice note to end on.

Bean and Barley Soup
Most people have a favourite recipe from mom. This is one of mine.

Bring 16 cups (4 L) stock to a boil. Add 1 cup (250 mL) barley, washed and drained, and 1 cup (250 mL) large dried lima beans. Chop and add celery, onion and carrots. Season with a pinch of thyme, basil and ground pepper.

Cook slowly for 1 to 1 1/2 hours until beans are tender. If too thick, add water.

For a delicious meatless thick pea soup, use 2 cups (500 mL) dried green split peas instead of beans and barley.

Serve soup with warmed whole-grain buns and a green salad. Delight the family with yogurt-topped baked apples for dessert.

Marvelous Italian Minestrone
Add a cornucopia of seasonal vegetables to gently simmering broth. The longest-cooking ones—potatoes, carrots, onions—go in first. The fastest-cooking kinds—leeks, green beans, zucchini—go in last. Boost your nutrition by adding pasta, beans or rice. Use your biggest soup pot. Minestrone tastes even better reheated—and it freezes beautifully.

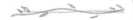

Soup "cans" to remember

- You *can* do away with added oil, butter or margarine, even if a recipe calls for it. Try it without and see if you notice any difference.
- You *can* still enjoy creamed and thickened soups the Heart-Smart way. Thicken them with potatoes, beans, noodles, rice or puréed vegetables, or use low-fat milk.
- You *can* easily make your own stock and control its salt and fat content. To make handy stock "cubes" for cooking, boil broth down to concentrate flavour. Strain. Freeze in ice cube trays.
- Canned broth may contain fat and salt. To remove fat, refrigerate the can so that the fat solidifies on the surface. Look for low-salt varieties.

Pizza pleasures

Keep the basics in your kitchen and you can put together a terrific pizza faster than it takes to order out. It's a lot cheaper too. Keep an eye on the amount of fat you add by using smaller quantities of lower-fat mozzarella cheese, avoiding high-fat meat choices and choosing lower-fat pizza shells.

Pizza with pizzaz

For the base, use pita bread or packaged whole-wheat pizza shells. Choose the mini-pitas and let your family build custom pizzas. Spread with bottled or homemade tomato sauce (see page 50). Top with vegetables—almost anything goes. Sliced tomatoes, mushrooms or peppers, artichoke hearts, broccoli florets, minced sun-dried tomatoes, roasted vegetables (see page 70). Highlight with a sprinkling of chopped olives, capers or anchovies.
Sprinkle lightly with lower-fat mozzarella cheese.
Add freshly ground pepper plus a sprinkling of dried basil or rosemary.
Bake in hot oven for 10 minutes. Enjoy a big green salad on the side.

The End!

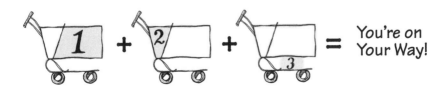

You're on Your Way!

Health Check™...tells you it's a healthy choice

Healthy eating is very important for good health. For more than a decade, the Heart and Stroke Foundation's HeartSmart™ materials and programs have helped consumers make healthy eating a part of their daily routine. We're proud to add *HeartSmart Nutrition* to our growing collection of consumer publications such as the Lighthearted and HeartSmart™ cookbooks, which have sold over 1.5 million copies!

And now we're excited to tell you about Health Check, a food information program that can help you make wise food choices at the grocery store. A national poll told us that 92% of Canadians think a standard on-pack symbol would help you, and that 92% of Canadians trust the Heart and Stroke Foundation to run such a program. Since most food purchase decisions are made in mere seconds right in the store, we're glad to be there with you, helping you make those healthy choices more often with Health Check, our made-in-Canada food information program.

How does Health Check Work?

Every food product participating in the program displays the *Health Check logo* and an *explanatory message* describing briefly how the food is part of healthy eating. It is also displays a *detailed Nutrition Facts table*. See the example below:

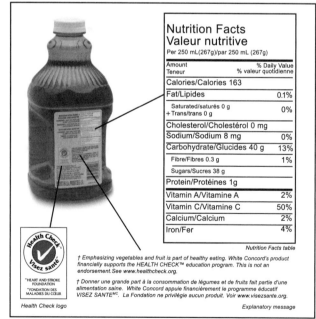

Nutrition Facts / Valeur nutritive	
Per 250 mL(267g)/par 250 mL (267g)	
Amount / Teneur	% Daily Value / % valeur quotidienne
Calories/Calories 163	
Fat/Lipides	0.1%
Saturated/saturés 0 g + Trans/trans 0 g	0%
Cholesterol/Cholestérol 0 mg	
Sodium/Sodium 8 mg	0%
Carbohydrate/Glucides 40 g	13%
Fibre/Fibres 0.3 g	1%
Sugars/Sucres 38 g	
Protein/Protéines 1g	
Vitamin A/Vitamine A	2%
Vitamin C/Vitamine C	50%
Calcium/Calcium	2%
Iron/Fer	4%

Nutrition Facts table

† *Emphasizing vegetables and fruit is part of healthy eating. White Concord's product financially supports the HEALTH CHECK™ education program. This is not an endorsement. See www.healthcheck.org.*

† *Donner une grande part à la consommation de légumes et de fruits fait partie d'une alimentation saine. White Concord appuie financièrement le programme éducatif VISEZ SANTÉ^MC. La Fondation ne privilégie aucun produit. Voir www.visezsante.org.*

"HEART AND STROKE FOUNDATION"
"FONDATION DES MALADIES DU CŒUR"

Health Check logo   *Explanatory message*

Health Check is based on Canada's Food Guide to Healthy Eating and promotes healthy eating in general, not just heart-healthy eating. Foods that display the Health Check logo meet specific nutrient criteria. There are different criteria for different food categories, depending on the important nutrient components of each food. For example, the criteria for bread focus on fat and fibre, whereas the criteria for milk products focus on fat and calcium. In a number of food categories, such as plain vegetables and fruit (fresh and frozen), all foods fit.

Participation in the program is voluntary. Companies follow a five-step process, from application to product review to new packaging, final licensing and fee payment. The Foundation applies a modest fee to run the program on a not-for-profit basis. Fees help cover the costs of administration, nutritional review, educational and promotional materials, technical support and the detailed Internet site. In addition, the Foundation conducts annual checks on selected participating products to ensure that they continue to meet the program criteria.

Although the presence of the logo assures you that the product is a healthy choice, the simple absence of the logo does not mean that the product is not. Some companies will opt not to participate. Products that do not display a Health Check logo may also be wise choices. If the Health Check logo is not present, look to the Nutrition Facts table to assist you in making purchasing decisions. The information you learn from reading this book will be helpful in understanding the food labels, and in making your final choices.

How will Health Check help you?

Health Check will simplify your shopping experience. You can be confident that the Heart and Stroke Foundation has reviewed any food bearing the Health Check logo, and that it is part of a healthy diet. The message, right on the package, will explain briefly how the product is part of healthy eating, reinforcing your ability to make healthy choices more often.

Look to the Nutrition Facts table, which under Canadian law is now mandatory on all packaging and will be introduced over the next three to five years, for additional nutrient information. We are also confident that a broader array of healthy choices will be presented in your grocery store! Manufacturers are keen to rise to the Health Check challenge and many will offer products that they have reformulated to fit Health Check's nutrient criteria. Imagine more delicious choices for healthier Canadians. That's when we all win!

Visit www.healthcheck.org or call your provincial Heart and Stroke Foundation office toll-free at 1-888-473-4636.

Health Check Participants!

Look for these brands displaying the Health Check logo in your grocery store. For more information about Health Check, and for a current list of participating companies, visit the Internet site at http://www.healthcheck.org.

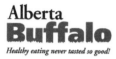
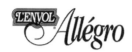

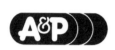

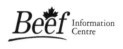

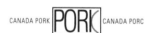
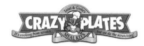
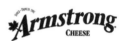

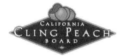
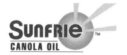

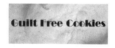
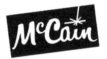
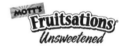

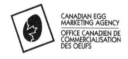

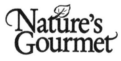
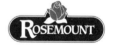

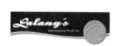

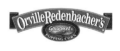

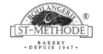

Cheerios

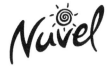

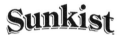
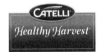
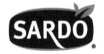

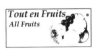

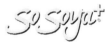

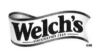

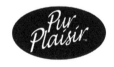

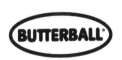

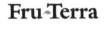

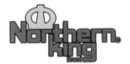

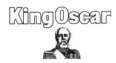

The Heart and Stroke Foundation of Canada and Ramona Josephson recognize the participation of the above-named participants in the Health Check program. This recognition does not constitute an endorsement by either the Heart and Stroke Foundation or Ramona Josephson of any of the participants' products.

Where foods fit in the total nutrition picture
according to Canada's Food Guide to Healthy Eating

NUTRIENTS	GRAIN PRODUCTS	VEGETABLES & FRUIT	MILK PRODUCTS	MEAT & ALTERNATIVES
Protein	Protein	—	Protein	Protein
Fat	—	—	Fat	Fat
Carbohydrate	Carbohydrate	Carbohydrate	Carbohydrate	—
Fibre	Fibre	Fibre	—	—
VITAMINS				
Thiamin	Thiamin	Thiamin	—	Thiamin
Riboflavin	Riboflavin	—	Riboflavin	Riboflavin
Niacin	Niacin	—	—	Niacin
Folic acid	Folic acid	Folic acid	—	Folic acid
Vitamin B12	—	—	Vitamin B12	Vitamin B12
Vitamin C	—	Vitamin C	—	—
Vitamin A	—	Vitamin A	Vitamin A	—
Vitamin D	—	—	Vitamin D	—
MINERALS				
Calcium	—	—	Calcium	—
Iron	Iron	Iron	—	Iron
Zinc	Zinc	—	Zinc	Zinc
Magnesium	Magnesium	Magnesium	Magnesium	Magnesium

Source: Using the Food Guide, Health and Welfare Canada, 1992

My Four Steps to Estimating Your Personal Fat Budget

I use these four simple steps to determine an individual's personal fat budget. Try it!

1. Find your desirable body weight by using the range in the BMI chart (below):
Desirable body weight = _____ kg

2. Calculate how many calories you need by multiplying your desirable weight by your activity factor:
If you are sedentary, multiply your desirable weight by 30.
If you are moderately active, multiply your desirable weight by 35.
If you are *very* active, multiply your desirable weight by 40.
Desirable body weight _____ kg X
_____ calories per kg = _____ calories

3. Calculate your fat budget in grams:
Divide the calories needed per day (Step 2) by 30.
_____ calories ÷ 30 = _____ grams of fat

4. Calculate your fat budget in teaspoons:
Divide your fat budget grams (Step 3) by 5.
_____ grams of fat ÷ 5 = _____ teaspoons of fat

Your Personal Fat Budget is _____ **teaspoons of fat per day.**

Body Mass Index Chart

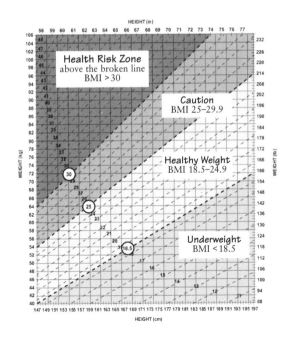

Source:
Health and Welfare
Canada. *Promoting
Healthy Weights:
A Discussion Paper.*
Ottawa: Minister of Supply
and Services Canada, 1988.

Fats and heart health

SATURATED FATS: tend to raise blood cholesterol. Usually solid at room temperature. Reduce your intake of these fats.

Key sources: meat, poultry, milk products (except skim milk products), butter, lard, tropical oils (palm, palm kernel and coconut) which are found in foods such as baked goods and other convenience foods.

MONOUNSATURATED FATS: help to lower blood cholesterol. Usually liquid at room temperature.

Key sources: olive oil, canola oil, avocado, olives, and nuts such as almonds, pistachios, pecans, hazelnuts and cashews.

POLYUNSATURATED FATS: help to lower blood cholesterol. Usually liquid at room temperature, they contain essential fatty acids that your body cannot manufacture.

Key sources: vegetable oils like safflower, sunflower, corn, and soybean, most nut oils, nuts such as walnuts, pine nuts, Brazil nuts and chestnuts, sunflower seeds, sesame seeds and fish.

OMEGA-3 FATTY ACIDS: a group of polyunsaturated fats. May help to lessen the risk of heart disease and stroke by reducing blood clotting and making platelets less likely to stick together.

Key sources: fatty fish such as salmon, trout and mackerel; canola, soy and flaxseed oils; and walnuts.

HYDROGENATION: a process in which hydrogen is added to liquid vegetable oil, changing it into a solid, which is more saturated and has a longer shelf life.

Key sources: vegetable shortening and other foods made with vegetable shortening such as cookies, crackers, chips and other packaged foods, some peanut butter and many but not all margarines.

TRANS FATTY ACIDS: created during the process of hydrogenation. They have been shown to raise blood cholesterol levels. Technically unsaturated fats, they act more like saturated fats.

Key sources: vegetable shortening and other foods made with vegetable shortening such as cookies, crackers, chips and other packaged foods, some peanut butter and many but not all margarines.

Figuring out the percentage of fat in a food

To calculate how many calories in a food come from fat:

1. Multiply the number of grams of fat by 9 (1 gram = 9 calories)—if a serving has 5 grams of fat, then 45 calories come from fat.
2. Divide the number of calories from fat by the number of calories in the serving. If the total calories of the serving are 90, then 45 ÷ 90 = 0.5.
3. Multiply the number by 100 to get the percentage—0.5 x 100 = 50% calories from fat.

Remember:

1. The 30% figure applies to your overall diet—what you eat over a day or a week. You don't need to figure it out for every individual food.
2. The percentage of fat calories is not as important if you eat the foods very rarely or if you don't eat much.
3. The percentage of fat calories is not as important when the food is low in calories.

Sources of cholesterol

Health and Welfare Canada—Nutrition Recommendations 1990 suggests that "reducing the cholesterol intake of the population towards 300 mg/day or less would be beneficial in the long term for the reduction of mortality from coronary artery disease."

Here are some common sources of dietary cholesterol. Remember, cholesterol is found only in foods from animals and fish.

mg cholesterol	quantity	source
631	3.5 oz (100 g)	chicken liver
432	2 large	eggs
415	3.5 oz (100 g)	beef liver
344	"	kidney
125–160	"	shrimp
70–120	"	beef, pork, lamb; most cuts
75–100	"	poultry
87	"	crab
78	"	lobster
53	"	clams
48	"	scallops
47	"	oysters
47	1.5 oz (45 g)	cheddar cheese made from whole milk
35	1 cup (250 mL)	milk, whole
31	1 tbsp (15 mL)	butter
10	1 cup (250 mL)	milk, 1% fat

Nutrient content claims

A nutrient content claim describes the amount of nutrient in a food. It is based on the reference amount and a serving of stated size.

Calorie claims

What it says	What it means
Calorie-free	less than 5 calories
Low in calories	40 calories or less
Reduced or lower in calories	at least 25% less energy
Source of calories	at least 100 calories

Fat claims

What it says	What it means
Fat-free	less than 0.5 g fat
Low in fat	3 g or less fat
Reduced or lower in fat	at least 25% less fat
100% fat-free	less than 0.5 g fat per 100 g, no added fat and "free of fat"
(naming the %) fat-free	"low in fat"

Saturated fatty acids

What it says	What it means
Saturated fatty acid-free	less than 0.2 g saturated fatty acids and less than 0.2 g trans fatty acids
Low in saturated fatty acids	2 g or less saturated fatty acids and trans fatty acids combined and 15% or less energy from saturated fatty acids plus trans fatty acids
Reduced or lower in saturated fatty acids	at least 25% less saturated fatty acids, and trans fatty acids not increased

Trans fatty acids

What it says	What it means
Free of trans fatty acids	less than 0.2 g trans fatty acids and "low in saturated fatty acids"
Reduced or lower in trans fatty acid	at least 25% less trans fatty acids, and saturated fatty acids not increased

Polyunsaturated fatty acids

What it says	What it means
Source of omega-3 polyunsaturated fatty acids	0.3 g or more omega-3 polyunsaturated fatty acids
Source of omega-6 polyunsaturated fatty acids	2 g or more omega-6 polyunsaturated fatty acids

Cholesterol

What it says	What it means
Cholesterol-free	less than 2 mg cholesterol and "low in saturated fatty acids"
Low in cholesterol	20 mg or less cholesterol and "low in saturated fatty acids"
Reduced or lower in cholesterol	at least 25% less cholesterol and "low in saturated fatty acids"

Sodium

What it says	What it means
Sodium-free or salt-free	less than 5 mg sodium or salt
Low in sodium or salt	140 mg or less sodium or salt
Reduced or lower in sodium or salt	at least 25% less sodium or salt
No added sodium or salt	no salt or other sodium salts added during processing
Lightly salted	at least 50% less added sodium or salt

Sugars

What it says	What it means
Sugar-free	less than 0.5 g sugars and (except chewing gum) "free of energy"
Reduced or lower in sugar	at least 25% less sugars
No added sugar	no sugars added in processing or packaging, including ingredients that contain added sugars or ingredients that functionally substitute for added sugars (e.g., concentrated fruit juice) and sugars not increased through some other means

Fibre

What it says	What it means
Source of fibre	2 g or more fibre or of each identified fibre
High fibre source	4 g or more fibre or of each identified fibre
Very high source of fibre	6 g or more fibre or of each identified fibre
More fibre	at least 25% more fibre and at least 2 g fibre

Light

What it says	What it means
Light	"reduced in energy" or "reduced in fat"

Sources of dietary fibre

Very high source

More than 6 g/serving

1/3 cup (75 mL)	some concentrated bran cereals (check label)
1/2 cup (125 mL)	baked beans in tomato sauce
1/2 cup (125 mL)	cooked kidney beans

High source

More than 4 g/serving

1/4 cup (50 mL)	100% wheat bran
1/2 cup (125 mL)	cooked dried peas, lima beans, navy beans
1 cup	cooked wild rice

Source

More than 2 g/serving

1/2 cup (125 mL)	some flaked bran cereals (check label)
1/4 cup (50 mL)	wheat germ
2 slices	whole-wheat bread
1/2 cup (125 mL)	cooked lentils
1 cup (250 mL)	cooked brown rice
1/2 cup (125 mL)	corn, peas, spinach, brussels sprouts
1 medium	potato with skin
1/2 cup (125 mL)	berries, cantaloupe
1/2 medium	pear
1 medium	apple, banana, orange, broccoli, carrots
2	prunes
3 tbsp (50 mL)	raisins

Heart-Healthy Cookbooks
from the Heart and Stroke Foundation of Canada

The Lighthearted Cookbook by Anne Lindsay (Key Porter), 2003.

Anne Lindsay's Lighthearted Everyday Cooking by Anne Lindsay (John Wiley & Sons Canada Ltd.), 2002.

Simply HeartSmart™ Cooking by Bonnie Stern (Random House of Canada), 1994.

More HeartSmart™ Cooking by Bonnie Stern (Random House of Canada), 1997.

HeartSmart™ Cooking for Family and Friends by Bonnie Stern (Random House of Canada), 2000.

HeartSmart™ Chinese Cooking by Stephen Wong (Douglas & McIntyre), 1996.

HeartSmart™ Flavours of India by Krishna Jamal (Douglas & McIntyre), 1998.

Index